The 17 Day Diet

About the Author

Dr Michael Rafael Moreno, better known as Dr Mike, is a graduate of the University of California at Irvine and Hahnemann Medical School (now Drexel University). Following his residency at Kaiser Permanente in Fontana, California, Dr Mike moved to San Diego, where he now practises family medicine and sits on the board of the San Diego Chapter of the American Academy of Family Physicians.

In 2008 Dr Mike launched 'Walk with Your Doc' (http://www.walkwith yourdoc.com), which he participates in every Tuesday and Thursday morning before his workday begins. The programme began when Dr Mike offered to walk with a patient to motivate her to exercise, and has since grown into a thriving community.

Dr Mike takes pride in being viewed not only as a doctor, but also as a friend and confidant.

'We've all pledged, promised and bullied ourselves to eat better and exercise more, but so many times even the best intentions fall short', Dr Mike says. 'I incorporate healthy habits into my work and home life, and you can too.'

The 17 Day Diet

*A Doctor's Plan Designed
for Rapid Results*

DR MIKE MORENO

SIMON &
SCHUSTER

London · New York · Sydney · Toronto

A CBS COMPANY

Disclaimer: This publication is intended to provide helpful and informative material. It is not intended to diagnose, treat, cure or prevent any health problem or condition, nor is intended to replace the advice of a doctor. No action should be taken solely on the contents of this book. Always consult your doctor or qualified health-care professional on any matters regarding your health and before adopting any suggestions in this book or drawing inferences from it.

The author and publisher specifically disclaim all responsibility for any liability, loss or risk, personal or otherwise, which incurred as a consequence, directly or indirectly, from the use or application of any contents of this book.

Any and all product names referenced within this book are the trademarks of their respective owners. None of these owners have been sponsored, authorised, endorsed or approved by this book. Always read all information provided by the manufacturers' labels before using their products. The author and publisher are not responsible for claims made by manufacturers. The statements made in this book have not been evaluated by the Food Standards Agency..

First published in Great Britain in 2011 by Simon & Schuster UK Ltd
A CBS COMPANY

7 9 10 8

Simon & Schuster UK Ltd
1st Floor
222 Gray's Inn Road
London
WC1X 8HB

www.simonandschuster.co.uk

Simon & Schuster Australia
Sydney

A CIP catalogue copy for this book is available
from the British Library.

ISBN: 978-0-85720-702-9

Designed by Leigh McLellan Design
Printed and bound by CPI Group (UK) Ltd, Croydon, CR0 4YY

Contents

* * * * * * * * * *

Dedication

I dedicate this book to my family and friends who have
supported me and my dreams, but most importantly
to my mother and father who always encouraged and
supported me. They placed a big emphasis on education,
and instilled in me the importance of hard work and helping
others. I would also like to thank my patients for providing
me with the motivation to think outside the box, in hopes
of making this world a healthier happier place.

Acknowledgements

I feel a deep sense of gratitude to Maggie Greenwood-Robinson. Without her persistence and endless hours of dedication to this project the book you are holding in your hands may not have been written. I'd also like to thank the many people involved in putting the programme and its support materials together.

My hope is that this book will help make the world a healthier and happier place. It's never too late to be fit and fabulous!

PART I

· · · · · · · · · · · · · · ·

The 17 Day Diet

1

Just Give Me 17 Days

I can personally sum up the 17 Day Diet in two words: fast results.

Depending on your weight when you start out and your metabolism, you might expect to lose up to 4.5 kg to 5.4 kg (10 to 12 lb) in the first 17 days. Of course, the further you are from your ideal weight, the more you'll lose initially.

Let's be realistic: when you start a diet, you want to see results straight away in how you look and feel. That's because our society is geared towards the immediate: we want things and we want them now. The same is true of weight loss. We get impatient when the pounds don't come off fast enough to meet our expectations. It seems much easier to give up than to go on.

This diet is designed to produce quick results, not because it starves you down to size but because its carefully designed balance of food and exercise adjusts your body metabolically so that you burn fat, day in and day out.

Also important is that the weight-reduction portion of this diet is limited to just 17 days at a time so that you aren't demoralised by the thought of endless months of dieting.

Nor are you apt to plateau like you often do on other diets. The 17 Day Diet keeps your body and metabolism guessing. I call this 'body confusion'. With each 17 Day Cycle, you're changing your calorie count and the foods you eat. By varying these things you prevent your body adapting. The scale is less likely to get stuck. The added bonus: you'll never get bored. And it's fun watching those pounds melt off. So confusion is good!

At the end of 17 days, you'll go on to a second 17-day Cycle, then a third and finally enter the Weight-stabilisation Cycle of the diet in which you get to eat a greater variety of foods, including your favourite foods *within reason*. (I don't want you to get too cosy with the all-you-can-eat buffets again.)

I already know what you're thinking: is it possible to shed pounds swiftly yet safely? If done right, without sacrificing good nutrition, the answer is yes.

Despite what many nutritionists have preached for years, rapid weight-loss diets can be healthy if done correctly and can work wonders on reducing pounds and inches in just days. Brand-new research suggests that the faster you take weight off, the longer you keep it off. Now that's a reason for dieters everywhere to rejoice. Plus, if you're too embarrassed by a recent weight increase or have just gained a noticeable 3.5 kg (8 lb) after a holiday weekend or an ice cream binge, this diet can get you back on track fast.

The 17 Day Diet thus gives your body the perfect kick-start, the kind of quick drop in weight that gives you a powerful mental boost. My whole focus is to get you thin as soon as I can. When I do, just think, you'll no longer have to move around hauling the equivalent of two 20 kg (45 lb) bags of cement on your body. The button of your jeans will no longer pop out and ping off the wall. You'll no longer have to wear plus-sized clothing with those expandable waistlines. This diet will make you slim, healthy and curvy, and I won't make you slurp your way to a thinner you, or follow some hardcore exercise regime used by the Royal Navy.

However, you do have to accept that this won't be a pleasure diet. You've got to stop eating unhealthy stuff. You've got to eat vegetables, fruits and

DOCTOR, CAN YOU PLEASE TELL ME ?

But won't a lot of the weight I lose be water weight?

Yes! And that's awesome, because water is weight too. Never dismiss those extra pounds as only 'water weight'; this is a self-defeating attitude. Cosmetically, water weight can hide fat loss and be particularly frustrating. Healthwise, fluid retention can put a strain on your heart. When your body holds water, this means there's more water in your blood. Your heart has to work harder to pump all that extra volume. Once all that excess fluid has disappeared, so will bloating and puffiness. You'll start looking visibly thinner in three or four days. And chances are, you'll feel much lighter and be more motivated to watch what you eat.

lean meat. I'm not going to ask you to probe your inner eater and uncover hidden emotional reasons for why you're fat. However, I am going to ask you to keep your portions down, cut your intake of fatty, sugary, salty foods, and move your bum. You won't be faint with hunger or found in the kitchen at midnight, feeding on sugar-laden cereals and biscuits. You can do this because anyone can do anything for 17 days.

The beauty of this programme is that you won't get discouraged or bored by the prospect of staying on a diet for what seems like for ever. It can yield results that will stand the test of time just as well as those long-term diets that emphasise depressingly slow incremental drops in weight. You'll love the fact that in seven, ten or 17 days, you'll be slimmer. And chances are, you'll feel a lot lighter and have an absurd amount of energy.

The 17 Day Diet is do-able and easy – unlike so many other diets, which are slightly less complicated than the checklist for a shuttle launch.

SCIENCE SAYS: Slow Isn't Necessarily Better

Conventional wisdom says that rapid weight loss leads to rapid weight regain. However, a new generation of science shows that slow isn't necessarily better.

Shape Up the Fast Way. A 2010 study from the University of Florida suggests that the key to long-term weight loss and maintenance is to lose weight quickly, not gradually. Amongst 262 obese middle-aged women, fast weight losers were those who shed more than 900 g (2 lb) a week. Compared to more gradual losers, fast weight losers lost more weight overall, maintained their weight loss longer and were less likely to put weight back on. The findings were published in the *International Journal of Behavioral Medicine*.

Trim Belly Fat. We pack on two forms of belly fat. One type collects around internal organs (also known as visceral fat). This type of fat raises blood pressure and cholesterol levels, and increases the risk of diabetes, Alzheimer's disease and even some cancers. Visceral fat is far more sinister than fat elsewhere in the body.

The other type sits just under the skin and is known as subcutaneous abdominal fat. It causes a hard-to-get-rid-of belly pouch. In a Finnish study published in the *International Journal of Obesity and Related Metabolic Disorders*, a rapid weight loss diet followed for 6 weeks trimmed visceral abdominal fat by 25 per cent and abdominal subcutaneous fat by 16 per cent.

So can you just give me 17 days?

If you can, congratulations! You won't be disappointed.

What Lies Ahead?

So what is this 17 Day Diet? I'll go into depth in the next few chapters, but as a very quick summary, the 17 Day Diet is a fun, fantastic way of eating designed to take off weight quickly. It's based on some very simple principles, one of which is eating foods that favour fat-burning and are friendly to your digestive system.

I want to emphasise that excess weight is always a sign of nutritional and metabolic imbalance. Contrary to popular assumption, it's not strictly a question of how much exercise you do or how much food you eat. Rather, it's also a question of what types of foods are eaten, and how they are digested, assimilated and metabolised. If any of these components of good nutrition are compromised, then the body will not be adequately nourished at the cellular level, metabolic function will be impaired and toxins will accumulate. Thus, to lose weight fast we need to optimise digestion and metabolism. That's what the 17 Day Diet does.

Trust me, you'll love the rapid loss of a few pounds so much that you'll decide to keep on going. After the first 17 days, there's another 17 days and another – three total Cycles and a maintenance Cycle in which you get to eat whatever the heck you want, mainly on weekends. Here's an overview:

Quick and Easy Overview of the 17 Day Diet

Cycles	Purpose
Cycle 1: Accelerate (17 days)	To promote rapid weight loss by improving digestive health. It helps clear sugar from the blood to boost fat-burning and discourage fat storage.
Cycle 2: Activate (17 days)	To reset your metabolism through a strategy that involves increasing and decreasing your caloric consumption to stimulate fat-burning and to help prevent plateaus.
Cycle 3: Achieve (17 days)	To develop good eating habits through the re-introduction of additional foods and move you closer to your goal weight.

Cycle 4: Arrive (ongoing)	To keep you at your goal weight through a programme of eating that lets you enjoy your favourite foods on weekends, whilst eating healthily during the week.

Once we're through with all the basics, I'm going to talk to you about how to follow the diet. I can't wait to show you all of its wonderful components and start you on your way to looking fit and fabulous. Take it one step at a time so that you don't get overwhelmed.

Your Appointment with Me

I might as well take a moment here to introduce myself. I'm a family practice doctor in the US. Under America's health insurance system, most people go first to a doctor like me for all complaints, from infections to chronic illnesses. I love the diversity of family practice. One moment, I'm treating an 18-year-old man with the flu; the next, a 90-year-old woman with joint pain.

I became a doctor for the reasons most people do – because I wanted to save lives, pure and simple. In my heart of hearts, I believe a doctor is so much more than a person who dispenses medication or marks off symptoms like a checklist at a sushi bar. He or she should treat the whole person. I make it a point to get to know each patient as a person before I put a stethoscope to his or her chest.

You can spend quite a lot of time in the waiting room, especiallly if you go to a walk-in clinic. In fact, you can spend more time in a waiting room than the person who decorated it. It's almost like going to a restaurant and being told that, even though you have a reservation, you have to sit at the bar for a while. The only difference is that in the doctor's surgery no one offers you a cocktail.

The next time you have to wait for what seems like an eternity, do some fun things to pass the time. Make collages from the magazines and sell them to other patients. Or peel off all the wallpaper without disturbing any of the artwork or posters.

I do things differently in my surgery. My patients don't need to wait for ever. My patients often don't even sit on the examining table when I talk to them. I sit on the examining table and they get the comfortable chair. The butcher paper upholstering the examining table is wonderful to draw on. Sometimes I hop off the table and start drawing pictures of organs to explain things to patients.

I'm responsible for 2,000 patients, though not all in one day. Many of them are women, and 80 per cent of my new patients are overweight. Most know it. One of the things I've always found interesting is that my patients often come in with a complaint of back pain, or knee pain or just plain old fatigue. Before I can get a word out, they say, 'I know it's because I'm fat'. Patients are smart.

Ever since I became a doctor, I've always been concerned with prevention. Prevention is the doorway to longevity. I hate using medications to treat problems that can be fixed with simple changes in lifestyle.

A good example is a patient I'll call Sharon, aged 60. Sharon has type 2 diabetes. When I first started seeing her she was taking oral diabetes medication. Once she changed to a healthier diet and started walking regularly with a friend she was able to get off all her medicines. What a triumph that was!

Then about a year ago Sharon came in for her regular appointment. We reviewed the results of her latest blood work. Her sugars were through the roof. A test that reflects a patient's blood sugar over the past 90 days was suddenly out of range.

What on earth had happened?

As we talked, Sharon told me that she no longer had a walking partner so she stopped exercising altogether.

'I'll walk with you!' I volunteered. I couldn't bear to see her health slip. So I became her walking partner. Before long, others joined us. Our walking group became affectionately known as *Walk with Your Doc* and has swelled to sometimes more than 50 people of all ages. We walk every Tuesday and Thursday morning without fail. I love it because I thrive on helping people live full, healthy, active lives.

Of course, a huge part of prevention is weight management. You see, the death toll racked up by heart disease, high blood pressure, stroke, diabetes and all the other fat-related diseases is scary. Studies even associate obesity with poor immune function. That makes overweight people more susceptible to infections and cancer. Obesity will kill far more Americans each year than any terrorist would dare dream of taking out.

Everybody knows this. I'm just bringing it up again to remind you that tubs of ice cream and large packets full of crisps are not worth shortening your life over.

We're already in so much trouble with trans fats, cheap sugars, excess sodium and unpronounceable additives jazzing up junk food – stuff that causes

DOCTOR, CAN YOU PLEASE TELL ME ?

Do I have to exercise whilst on the 17 Day Diet?

Yes, but I won't be asking you to sweat to golden oldies, pump it up or feel the burn. In other words – no over-exercising. Since you'll be scaling back on calories, you should do less exercising, or else you'll get too run down and sore, especially during the first two Cycles. However, I will ask you to do just 17 minutes a day of easy exercising such as walking.

The 17 Day Diet has a companion exercise DVD called the 17 Minute Workout that you can purchase from our website, www.the17daydiet.com. It's cardio-based and geared towards pure fat-burning.

So put down this book. Do this workout, or go outside and walk around your neighbourhood for 17 minutes. Then come back and pick up where you left off.

your arteries to clog up like rusty pipes. With everything plaguing a Western-style diet, I had to concentrate on creating a programme that would be safe, effective and produce quick but lasting results. People had to get the weight off, then learn how to keep it off. I didn't want to tell my patients to go on this diet or that diet because many diets out there are nutritionally unbalanced, hard to follow or just don't work fast enough to keep you motivated.

Thus, the 17 Day Diet evolved. It uses the latest medical knowledge on nutrition, foods and what the body needs for successful weight loss and good health.

Let me add here that you should check with your own doctor before starting this programme. Your doctor knows what's best for you. Based on my experience with my own patients, most people who have got out of shape over the years can follow the 17 Day Diet and do very well on it, though results can vary.

There Is More to Love about the 17 Day Diet ...

Whether you've got 10 pounds to lose or a hundred, being overweight is one of life's lesser joys. It affects every aspect of your life, maybe some things you never thought about. When you lose weight, practically everything in your life will change for the better. Let's talk about this now.

Get a Healthy Body

You're going to be focused on losing pounds and inches. Some days you might get a little discouraged if the scales don't move down fast enough, even though this diet does help prevent plateaus. However, there's absolutely nothing to be discouraged about. There are other wonderful things happening inside your body that won't be reflected on the scales, like your blood pressure, blood sugar and cholesterol decreasing.

Okay, I realise that right now you might not care about these things. You just want to slip into that sexy black number hanging in your wardrobe ... you know, the one that used to fit years ago. But it's important to understand that your weight and health are not separate issues. Being overweight is a symptom of being unhealthy. Focus on your weight and your health will improve – instantly. Consider what the results of various research studies say about the rather immediate effects of healthy nutrition on the body:

After 15 minutes: After the first morning of eating a healthy breakfast, your stomach's satiety signals have registered in your brain, and you feel full. The body's internal chemistry is at its most active first thing in the morning, so your breakfast is then used to the maximum. If you eliminated processed foods (white bread, sugary cereals) and substituted whole grains and lean proteins such as egg whites, along with fresh fruit, you should feel energetic and mentally alert after just one meal.

After 3 hours: Your artery linings are able to expand sufficiently to increase blood flow to the body's tissues and organs.

After 6 hours: The HDL (happy cholesterol) in your blood perks up and starts scouring LDL (lousy cholesterol) from the blood. You can think of LDLs as delivery lorries, depositing cholesterol in blood vessels, and HDLs as rubbish lorries, taking them back to the liver where they're broken down.

After 12 hours: Your body finally has an opportunity to burn the fat it has stored for energy because you've eliminated sugar. When you're eating a lot of sugar, your body is so busy processing the sugar that it doesn't have time to do its other job, which is to help the body burn fat. So guess what? The fat ends up hanging around.

After 16 hours: You get a restful night's sleep.

After 24 hours: You're 450 to 900 g (1 to 2 lb) lighter, because your body has begun to flush excess water and toxins from your system.

After 3 days: Once your body senses it's losing weight, its blood-related numbers (cholesterol, blood pressure, blood sugar) start travelling in a healthy direction.

After 1 week: Your cholesterol levels can drop significantly. Blood levels of important disease-fighting antioxidants such as vitamin C and vitamin E are higher. Your bowels are in better working order, and you should be at least 2.25 kg (5 lb) lighter.

After 2 weeks: You'll experience healthy drops in blood pressure if you've been diagnosed with hypertension. Expect to have lost up to 4.5 kg (10 lb) by now.

After 1 month: You won't have to filter out chunks of fast food from your blood any more. By now blood levels of LDL cholesterol can fall by nearly 30 per cent – a drop similar to that seen with some cholesterol-lowering medicines.

After 6 weeks: You've lost so much weight you can't buy new, smaller clothes fast enough. Yes, you should have lost quite a bit of weight (9 kg/20 lb is not unusual), and your blood cholesterol and triglyceride levels will be substantially improved.

After 12 weeks: Many significant health numbers – cholesterol, triglycerides (fat in the blood), blood pressure, glucose and insulin – should begin to, if not completely, normalise.

After 6 months: You'll feel healthier because your body will be retaining more vitamins and minerals. Because you reduced your sugar intake significantly over this period, insulin production will have normalised. So your risk of developing type 2 diabetes is reduced, as this can be linked to a larger intake of sugar. Your energy levels have improved dramatically because your body has gone through a detoxing process. You've probably reached your goal. The hardest work is over, and now it's time to learn how to eat to maintain your newly slender silhouette.

Pretty amazing what a good diet can do, right? Don't you want all of this? Be brutally honest here: if you really want something you'll find a way to get it. So if you find yourself saying, 'I didn't have time to prepare healthy food', let me ask you this: would you have found time if your life depended on it? Well, it does.

GET SKINNY SHORTCUT

Posture

Stand up straight. Not only does slouching make your tummy protrude, but it gives your core muscles an undeserved break. Standing erect, with the stomach held in, encourages the abs to work and can make you look slimmer naturally – and in an instant.

Get Sexy

When you're fit and in shape, you're much more datable. In one survey of 554 undergrads, researchers found that overweight women were less likely to date than their peers. What's more, you're marriage material if you're thin. Research shows that overweight women are significantly less likely to marry than are women of average weight, particularly if they were overweight as young adults.

Losing weight can do wonders for your sex life too. Researchers at Duke University in the US did a study of 187 extremely obese adults, who were asked about their sex lives before and after they lost weight. It turned out the proportion of women who did not feel sexually attractive fell from 68 per cent before they began a weight loss programme to 26 per cent a year later. There were similar decreases in the percentages of women who didn't want to be seen naked, had little sexual drive, avoided sexual encounters, had difficulty with sexual performance or didn't enjoy sex. Amongst men, sex improved in most of the categories, but the improvements were less dramatic, probably because there are a lot more appearance-related pressures on women.

The romantic world revolves around physical appearances. If you want a love life with great sex, lose the weight.

Get Richer

Get in shape and you can improve your financial shape – and the NHS's – too. It's considerably more expensive to be unfit than it is to be fit, mainly because you're sicker more often and medical expenses are higher. People who are overweight, and particularly those who are obese, are significantly more likely to have expensive-to-treat diseases such as diabetes, heart disease and cancer.

And whilst I'm at it, did you know your employment prospects will improve after you lose weight? It's true! People with weight problems sometimes don't get hired. In the job market, appearance counts for a lot. Employers think fat people are lazy, incompetent, slow-moving and might have poor attendance. Studies have shown that fat people are paid less than employees of average weight.

I hate fat discrimination. It's wrong. However, this is the world we live in. It's not going to change anytime soon, so get to grips with it. Lose weight and you won't have to deal with it.

Thin people look better, and, like it or not, get paid more. If you're trim and healthy, you don't have an absentee problem. You might even be more productive on the job. All of this helps your earning potential. So if you want to live well and make your mortgage or rent payment, get those pounds off.

If my message seems too blunt, I apologise for the delivery – but not for the content. I'm speaking out because I care. I just want you to get healthy and enjoy your life to the fullest.

LEAN 17: Are You Ready to Be a Total Hottie?

Take this quiz to see if you are ready to go on the 17 Day Diet. A successful and healthy weight loss requires the right frame of mind. Circle the answer that best describes your level of commitment.

1. When I think about starting the 17 Day Diet I feel excited.

   A. Yes   **B.** Somewhat   **C.** Unsure   **D.** Not at all

2. I feel that weight loss and fitness are very important.

   A. Yes   **B.** Somewhat   **C.** Unsure   **D.** Not at all

3. I am determined to eat more healthfully.

   A. Yes   **B.** Somewhat   **C.** Unsure   **D.** Not at all

4. I want to look better and feel sexier.

   A. Yes   **B.** Somewhat   **C.** Unsure   **D.** Not at all

5. I am willing to follow the food plans in this book.

   A. Yes   **B.** Somewhat   **C.** Unsure   **D.** Not at all

---

6. I will eat more fruits and vegetables.

   A. Yes   **B.** Somewhat   **C.** Unsure   **D.** Not at all

---

7. I will give up fizzy drinks, squash and sweets whilst following this diet.

   A. Yes   **B.** Somewhat   **C.** Unsure   **D.** Not at all

---

8. I will scale back on my alcohol intake.

   A. Yes   **B.** Somewhat   **C.** Unsure   **D.** Not at all

---

9. I will prepare more meals at home and eat out less frequently.

   A. Yes   **B.** Somewhat   **C.** Unsure   **D.** Not at all

---

10. I will increase my water intake.

    A. Yes   **B.** Somewhat   **C.** Unsure   **D.** Not at all

---

11. I am willing to cut back on starchy foods such as white bread, pasta and sugary breakfast cereals.

    A. Yes   **B.** Somewhat   **C.** Unsure   **D.** Not at all

---

12. I feel confident that I can stick to this plan for at least 17 days.

    A. Yes   **B.** Somewhat   **C.** Unsure   **D.** Not at all

---

13. I will eat at least 3 meals and 1 snack a day.

    A. Yes   **B.** Somewhat   **C.** Unsure   **D.** Not at all

---

14. I will not make excuses to sabotage myself.

    A. Yes   **B.** Somewhat   **C.** Unsure   **D.** Not at all

---

15. I can commit to exercising at least 17 minutes a day.

    A. Yes   **B.** Somewhat   **C.** Unsure   **D.** Not at all

---

16. I want to change my eating and health habits for life.

    A. Yes   **B.** Somewhat   **C.** Unsure   **D.** Not at all

---

17. I understand how diet, obesity and chronic illnesses are linked.

    A. Yes   **B.** Somewhat   **C.** Unsure   **D.** Not at all

Scoring: Give yourself a 3 for each A answer, a 2 for each B answer, a 1 for each C answer and 0 for each D answer. Add up your score.

0 to 17 points: Immediately re-evaluate your commitment to improving your health. If you don't act decisively now, serious health problems are on the horizon.

18 to 26 points: Go back over your answers and see what you need to improve. You may be taking some unnecessary risks with your health and should make an extra effort to change.

27 to 42 points: Re-examine your desire to go on the 17 Day Diet. What improvements can you make to boost your score? You need just a little bit more determination and commitment to be thinner and healthier.

43 to 51 points: You're ready to start the 17 Day Diet and enjoy success – congratulations!

You must believe you can do this. It doesn't matter how often you have failed in the past; your past does not equal your future. What matters now is focusing on what you want, identifying what you need to get it and taking action. Your health and happiness are important, so stand strong.

Review:

- The 17 Day Diet is a rapid weight loss plan designed to produce satisfying, lasting weight loss.
- Most people can expect to lose up to 4.5 to 6.8 kg (10 to 15 lb) during the first 17 days.
- Rapid weight loss plans have been shown in research to be effective in helping people keep their weight off.
- The 17 Day Diet works by improving digestive and metabolic health.
- The 17 Day Diet is organised into 4 Cycles, each working together to help your body reach its ideal weight and stabilise it there.
- Stay upbeat and positive. No matter what you weigh right now, stop putting yourself down. So much in your life can change for the better: your figure, health, relationships, financial stability and more.

6 REASONS Not to Worry About Being Fat

One of my patients joked recently about the pluses of her plus size: 'I can shoplift in my cleavage. And I don't have to ask my boyfriend, "Do I look fat in this?" I do.' That conversation got me thinking about some of the health advantages to being overweight. Although I don't recommend staying fat, there are some pluses to being a plus size. Here are six ways in which some padding can tip the scales in your favour.

Stronger Bones
A little meat on your frame can ward off osteoporosis, a condition of fragile bones that's less likely to occur in overweight women. Weight-bearing bones stay stronger.

Healthier Hearts and Lower Risk of Diabetes
Women with larger thighs have a lower risk of heart disease and early death, says a study in the *British Medical Journal.* Those with stick-thin legs face the greatest chance of developing heart disease. Why? Added lower-body muscle mass can promote a better metabolism. Also, a 2008 study published in *Cell Metabolism* found that the fat that accumulates around the thighs and hips, called subcutaneous fat, actually lowers risk of diabetes. Pear shapes, be proud.

Glowing Skin
Recent studies on twins have found that the sister with more weight was judged to have a more youthful look. A gaunt face can definitely add some years, so carrying an extra few pounds can help create a more youthful appearance. It may also help to fill out a few of those more significant wrinkles that tend to scream out 'ageing'!

Bigger Boobs
The more you weigh, the bigger they get. Breasts are made up of mostly fat, and any excess pounds practically go straight to your chest. Unfortunately, when you lose weight, boob flab is one of the first things to go.

Increased Fertility
Are you thinking of starting – or growing – your family? Underweight women were 72 per cent more likely to miscarry, reports a London study. More specifically, when leaner women conceived they had a much higher percentage of miscarrying within three months of pregnancy. However, those few extra pounds on overweight women actually proved to have the opposite effect on their pregnancy.

Faster Metabolism

It's not the skinny folks who have a fast metabolism; it's the overweight people! It takes more energy to operate anything bigger, so bigger people use more energy to do the same things that smaller people do. But metabolism isn't the only thing that determines weight; it's also how much you eat and exercise that matters.

Best Reason of All

People who are really out of shape, who start exercising, get fitter faster! The fact is your body wants to be in shape. It wants to be healthy. It wants to look good. It wants to be hot! So, the more out of shape you are, the faster your body will respond to your weight loss efforts.

2

Burn, Baby, Burn

ere's the part of the book in which I talk about how the 17 Day Diet works. Don't worry. I won't lapse into any mind-numbing 'doctor speak'. You know, medical terms that sound scarier than the disease, like cephalalgia (headache) or pneumonitis (lung inflammation). Most people have no idea what their doctors are saying. They could be giving them the latest medical research or the recipe for chocolate cheesecake in Latin. They couldn't tell.

I make a real effort to explain things in everyday terms. Sometimes, it's hard. I used to try to explain blood tests to patients in five minutes. It finally dawned on me that it took me eight years to understand this stuff, so I can't expect anyone to comprehend it during one surgery appointment. You don't need to study medical books to understand what doctors say anyway: just watch TV programmes and films.

Back to the topic of dieting: let me insert Rita's story here. If the subject of weight loss came up in conversation, she'd walk away. About 11 kg (25 lb) overweight, Rita was deep-down scared that she could get heavier if she didn't do something. But she just wasn't ready to confront the issue head-on. The idea of dieting and taking weight off slowly was frustrating, so she kept putting it off. But the 17 Day Diet appealed to her. It sounded do-able and quick – it is. Rita decided to have a go.

Here's what she said, 'I can't believe how well the 17 Day Diet works. I lost 10 pounds [4.5 kg] the first 17 days, and I feel so energetic. What gives? How does it work?'

Basically, Rita was hooked (in a positive way) and has used the diet to get to her goal and stay there. She stayed motivated.

I explained to Rita that for a diet and exercise programme to be successful, it must be safe, easy to follow and easy to stick to. It must have a certain balance of nutrients to activate fat-burning. It must generate results in a reasonable period of time. And it must help initiate a pattern of healthy habits that lead to lifelong weight control. The 17 Day Diet can help you accomplish all of this and more. What follows is a careful look at the elements that make this diet work.

What Do You Get to Eat on the 17 Day Diet?

First let me say, nutrition is too confusing, even for doctors. Everything is either good or bad for you. And that can change from moment to moment, each time a new bit of research is unveiled. Broccoli may double your life span this week, but next week it might be the end of you.

Several years ago, blueberries became the fruit of choice, being touted as the answer for everything from rejuvenating your brain to inhibiting the growth of cancer cells. Now they're being added to cosmetics. If they can prevent your brain ageing, why not put them in a skin cream? Maybe blueberries can stop wrinkles too.

I think you have to be living under a rock not to know that lean proteins, fruits, vegetables and small amounts of grains are naturally good for you. The 17 Day Diet is based on those foods. That's one reason why the diet isn't a fad; it's based on really healthy foods, the stuff we should all be eating anyway, but aren't.

With these wonderful foods, we get the body to store the good (health-building nutrients) and expel the bad (fat and toxins) by retraining your digestive system and your metabolism.

Many long and informative books have been written about nutrition and how it works in the body. For the purpose of this book I'll explain what you need to know about the nutrients your body needs to lose weight, and I'll do it in the clearest, most basic terms.

Enjoy Plenty of Protein

The 17 Day Diet is generous in protein. But I don't mean 27 eggs and 18 rashers of bacon washed down with the drippings. I mean lean foods such as chicken, fish, lean meats and other protein-rich foods.

Protein is a powerful fat torcher – for six reasons:

1. Digesting protein takes more energy (calories) than digesting carbs or fat does, so your body burns a few extra calories after eating protein.

2. Including ample protein in your diet spurs one of your body's fat-burning mechanisms: the production of the hormone glucagon. Glucagon signals your body to move dietary fat into your bloodstream and use it for energy rather than just store it.

3. Consuming enough protein helps you preserve lean muscle mass that might otherwise be sacrificed on a rapid weight loss diet. Of course, the more lean muscle you have, the more calories you burn, even at rest.

4. Eating protein helps keep your blood sugar on an even keel, so you don't get the shakes or drops in energy.

5. Having enough protein in your diet boosts your metabolism, and it does this by stepping up the action of your thyroid gland. (One of the main duties of the thyroid is to regulate metabolism.)

6. Including protein with meals helps tame your appetite so that you don't stuff yourself.

Venture into Vegetables

If you haven't eaten vegetables since you were 11, let's spend a second on this 'I hate vegetables' thing.

You hate all vegetables? There isn't one you like, no matter how it's prepared? If you eliminate all vegetables from your diet, you're giving up some very important nutrients and really narrowing your food options. Vegetables are loaded with fibre, vitamins and minerals. Shunning them is a bad idea. Why not learn to prepare them WITH herbs and spices to satisfy your taste?

Pardon my assumption, but I think you, like thousands of other people I've talked to, believe that to lose weight, you have to subsist on carrot and celery sticks. But the old 'carry around some celery sticks to munch on' mentality is gone forever. Aren't you relieved?

There are hundreds of different vegetables you can eat, even if you have to hide them in soups or pasta sauce. And you can happpily eat your way through a couple of bushels without gaining any weight. If you want to change your body and get leaner, stronger and healthier, you have to eat vegetables. A March 1999 study conducted by the Energy Metabolism Laboratory at Tufts University in the US found that the dieters who ate the widest variety of vegetables had the least amount of body fat. You need to eat vegetables if you want to get thin. Vegetables = thin. No vegetables = flabby.

Many of my patients have actually acquired a taste for fresh green salads with cucumbers, tomatoes, red onions, carrots, mushrooms and all sorts of veggies. Some of them have even turned themselves into health nuts who only dip their forks into the salad dressing to really slash caloric intake.

There are more benefits. Eat more vegetables and you will:

* Bubble with energy all day.
* Improve your digestion and elimination, because veggies are high in fibre. High-fibre foods control appetite and help prevent excess calories from being stored as fat.
* Have glowing skin. Your skin loves vitamins and minerals, and you get most of those nutrients from veggies.
* Help prevent major killers such as cancer and heart disease, because veggies are rich in disease-fighting antioxidants.

So yes, you heard me: eat your vegetables!

Give Up High-Sugar Fruits

Fruit may seem like a friendly diet food because it's low-fat, but here's an example of how having too much of a good thing can sabotage your diet. Certain fruits such as pineapple, watermelon and banana are high in sugar, and they don't promote fat loss. Too much sugar from any source can goad your body into converting more of what you eat into thigh-padding pounds.

I'm not going to ask you to shun all fruit. Just be moderate in how much you eat – two servings a day only. On the first two Cycles of the 17 Day Diet, you'll stick to berries, apples, oranges and grapefruit, which are lower in sugar. By eating like this a fruit tooth will replace the sweet one that rules your mouth.

Cut the Carbs

Carbohydrates are energy foods. Without them, you'd get foggy headed, grumpy and very tired, and no one will want to be around you. The low-carb diet craze deemed all carbs evil and fattening. People abandoned all forms of fruit, rice and pasta and ate mostly protein. The problem is you can only eat so much protein and fat before you start to get nauseated by it.

Yet, not all carbs are the same. There are bad ones – stuff made mostly out of sugar or over-refined such as white bread, white rice and white pasta. Sugar and sweets are the worst. Consider this: we are eating over twelve times the amount of sugar our great-grandparents consumed. That's roughly equivalent to 72.5 kg (160 lb) of sugar per person per year. Now, imagine filling up your living room or garage with 160 of those 450 g (1 lb) bags you buy at the supermarket. Really get a mental picture of it. Let's say you don't eat as much as others, and cut it in half. It's still a hefty pile, isn't it? You see, most people have no idea that they're eating so much sugar. Much of it is hidden in processed, packaged foods we eat, as well as in drinks.

Depending on which Cycle you are in on the 17 Day Diet, you get to eat good carbs: fruit, vegetables, whole grains – anything that hasn't been stripped of its nutrition.

So the type of carbs you eat is important. But so is the amount. You can go overboard on carbs, even the good kind, and this can be devastating to your natural metabolic processes. Therefore, the 17 Day Diet is low-to-moderate in carbohydrates.

Many people are walking around completely unaware that they may be 'carbohydrate sensitive'. When you get carbohydrate sensitive, your body can no longer burn fat effectively, and a good deal of the carbohydrates you eat are packed away as fat. Carbohydrate sensitivity occurs when:

- You habitually eat too much sugar and refined carbohydrates (bagels, pasta, sugary cereals and puddings, white rice and white bread). Unfortunately, this sensitivity increases with age. It can also lead to insulin resistance, a condition just shy of type 2 diabetes. In insulin resistance, cells don't recognise glucose any more, so glucose is barred from entering cells for energy. Your blood sugar tends to rise, you are more fatigued and you gain more weight mostly around your waist and chest area.

● You suffer from chronic stress. Our bodies deal with stress by raising cortisol levels, a hormone secreted from our adrenal glands. This in turn triggers the over-release of glucose and insulin into the bloodstream. The result is insulin resistance. To your physiology being under chronic stress is the same as if you ate cake all day long.

● You're a woman. While men burn carbohydrates for energy, women tend to store them as fat. This is especially true as women age. Menopausal women are more prone. They don't have enough oestrogen

---

CHECK UP: Are You Carbohydrate Sensitive?

Read through the statements below and circle 'yes' or 'no' depending on which response fits you best.

1.	I crave carbohydrates and sugary foods much of the time.	Yes	No
2.	I have been overweight for much of my life and have struggled to lose weight.	Yes	No
3.	I am a woman and over forty.	Yes	No
4.	I suffer from chronic or bouts of depression and compulsive overeating.	Yes	No
5.	I sometimes suffer from nervousness, irritability.	Yes	No
6.	When I eat sugar, I get tired and light-headed, and I don't think as clearly.	Yes	No
7.	I reach for carbohydrates over protein most or all of the time.	Yes	No
8.	My diet consists of a lot of processed foods such as white bread, pastas, sweets or sugary cereals.	Yes	No
9.	I don't exercise very much or at all.	Yes	No

If you answered 'yes' to three or more statements, you may be carbohydrate sensitive. Following the 17 Day Diet will help you by gradually reintroducing good carbs into your diet through each Cycle. Beans and lentils (pulses) do not raise blood sugar or insulin. Starchy vegetables – such as squash, corn, peas and yams – and fruits such as oranges and apples are also good and should be okay. So are brown rice, yams, oats and other high-fibre cereals. Limit your servings to no more than two a day. More on this in Cycle 3.

stores to deal with cortisol and its tendency to make the body store fat. Chalk it up to female biology.

Natural and unprocessed carbs are found in the 17 Day Diet in the vegetables and fruits allowed you. By Cycle 3 you'll get to introduce other carbs into the diet, including brown rice, oats, wholegrains, yams, potatoes and other natural, high-fibre carbs.

Choose Fats that Burn Fat

Fat in the diet has been blamed for many modern lifestyle diseases: obesity, heart disease, cancer, diabetes and hypertension. Not all fats are created equal, however. Most people know by now they should limit intake of saturated fats, found in animal foods, and avoid trans fats entirely. Processed foods are loaded with trans fats.

Polyunsaturated fats, found mostly in fish and vegetable oils, are what I call 'friendly fats'. They are credited with keeping your skin supple and youthful, reducing harmful levels of cholesterol, lowering high blood pressure, contributing to brain and eye development and a host of other health benefits almost akin to a panacea. They also promote weight loss because they keep you feeling fuller for a longer period of time. This keeps you from eating too many calories.

Omega-3 fatty acids, found in fish, boost your metabolism. Adding some weekly servings of fish high in omega-3s (salmon, tuna, mackerel or sardines), whilst reducing calories, helped overweight people lose more weight than reducing calories alone, according to a study published in the *American Journal of Clinical Nutrition*. The researchers concluded that the omega-3s helped subjects burn more calories. If you don't like fish, take 3 grams of fish oil supplements daily.

Vitamins from Food

You're better off getting your vitamins from food. The body absorbs them more easily, and you'll just feel healthier. Required by your body in tiny amounts, vitamins play important roles in the metabolism of carbohydrates, proteins and fats. The vitamins you need daily are found in the 17 Day Diet as follows:

Vitamin A: Green leafy vegetables, carrots, yams, fruits and eggs

Vitamin B-complex: Protein foods, whole grains, pulses, fruits and vegetables

DOCTOR, CAN YOU PLEASE TELL ME ?

Are there natural supplements I can take instead of medicines to help lower my cholesterol?

Yes! A strict diet can probably reduce your cholesterol by 10 to 15 per cent. Most doctors agree that diet works best when combined with cholesterol-reducing medications such as statin medicines. Statins can drop LDL and total cholesterol by as much as a third by inhibiting the production of cholesterol by the liver. But these medicines come with potential side effects, with the most common one being muscle aches. Other complaints include headaches, nausea, weakness, upset stomach and joint pain. I see these problems all the time.

Here's what I do for patients who can't tolerate statins but need to lower their cholesterol. I prescribe a combination of niacin (a B vitamin), fish oil and linseed (flaxseed) oil in these amounts:

- **Niacin:** 250 milligrams a day for two or more weeks until they experience no flushing, which is a common side effect of niacin. After two weeks, I increase their dose to 500 milligrams a day. Once they tolerate that dose well, I increase the dose again to 750 milligrams daily.
- **Fish oil:** 3 grams a day.
- **Linseed oil:** 1 tablespoon a day (this can be part of a salad dressing.)

All three substances are natural supplements you can purchase at a health food shop or your chemist. The combination works powerfully to lower cholesterol, but always check with your own doctor before starting supplements.

- *Vitamin C:* Fruits and vegetables
- *Vitamin D:* Low fat dairy foods, fish
- *Vitamin E:* Whole grains, green leafy vegetables and eggs

There's nothing wrong with taking a good multivitamin-mineral tablet daily.

Mighty Minerals

Minerals are amongst the heaviest substances ever, second only to Orson Welles. But of course, minerals don't make you heavy. They help you get thin, especially calcium, which may speed up the rate at which your body burns fat.

Like vitamins, minerals play a role in metabolism. But a major difference between the two nutrients is that minerals are constituents of bodily structures such as bone, cartilage and teeth, providing their hardness and strength. Whilst vitamins help manufacture these structures, they do not become part of the structures themselves.

The minerals you need daily are found in the 17 Day Diet as follows:

Iron: Meats, poultry, eggs, green leafy vegetables and fruits

Calcium: Yoghurt, salmon, green leafy vegetables and broccoli

Copper: Meats, shellfish.

Magnesium: Meats.

Phosphorus: Meats, poultry, fish

Potassium: Fruits and vegetables

Selenium: Wholegrains, fish and eggs

Zinc: Shellfish, meats, whole grains and vegetables

The Benefits of Bugs

Not the kind you swat or stomp, but the friendly bacteria called probiotics that live in your intestinal tract (sometimes referred to as your gut). You have a hundred trillion bacteria in your intestinal tract – ten times the number of cells – across three hundred to five hundred different species, and two hundred of these species can be lethal. This makes us more microbe than man. So you need to make sure you have enough of the good bacteria to ward off the bad.

There are actually two processes going on here. One is the good bacteria help your intestinal wall construct a barrier against the bad bacteria. The second is the good bacteria are like hostage negotiators you see on TV. They talk to the bad bacteria to keep them from starting a fight. The bad bacteria know the good guys mean business, so they drop their weapons and wave white flags.

The good guys do even more: probiotics may help people lose weight, according to lots of new research that adds to emerging evidence that part of the obesity problem might be an imbalance of bacteria in the intestinal tract.

Scientists are still exploring why, but many experts believe that people with certain communities of intestinal microbes may get more calories from their food and therefore pack on more fat than people with a different set of bugs. If you have a set of very, very efficient bacteria, they're going to extract every last bit of energy (calories) from what you eat. Manipulating these bacteria by diet or medications, you'd change how many calories you absorb. This may eventually become one approach to fighting obesity.

On the 17 Day Diet you'll enjoy foods that contain probiotics. These foods help your body digest foods and extract calories. Some types of probiotic foods include yoghurt, kefir, miso, tempeh and others.

Fluid Assets

While following the 17 Day Diet, you should drink eight 240 ml (8 fl oz) glasses of pure water daily. Drinking this amount of water is essential to weight loss.

First, it just takes up so much space in your tummy that you don't feel like eating anything else.

Second, water also helps your body metabolise stored fat. Your kidneys can't function properly without enough water. When kidneys don't work to capacity, some of their work is dumped on to the liver. One of the liver's primary functions is to metabolise stored fat into usable energy for the body, but if the liver has to do some of the kidneys' work, it can't operate at full capacity. As a result, it metabolises less fat and more fat remains stored in the body, and weight loss stops.

Water also helps the body get rid of waste during weight loss. During weight loss the body has a lot more waste to get rid of, and water helps flush it out.

Surprisingly, drinking an ample amount of water is the best treatment for fluid retention. When the body gets less water, it perceives this as a threat to survival and begins to hold on to every drop. Water is then stored outside the cells. This causes swollen feet, legs and hands. The best way to overcome the problem of water retention is to give your body what it needs: plenty of water. Only then will stored water be released.

So drink up. Before long, you'll be the skinniest person in the toilet.

BEWARE: Negative Water

The following fluids, which I call negative water, do not count towards your must-have daily allowance of water.

Coffee*

Tea*

Diet fizzy drinks or squash

Regular fizzy drinks or squash

Energy drinks

Juice

Sports drinks (dilute with water – ½ water and ½ sports drink
if you are an athlete and use these products)

Flavoured waters

*Coffee and tea are allowed on the 17 Day Diet, but do not count towards your 8 glasses of water.

Special Mention Fluids: Green Tea and Coffee

For added fat-loss benefits, another drink of choice is green tea, although it is technically a negative water. Certain natural chemicals called catechins in green tea increase fat-burning and stimulate thermogenesis, the calorie-burning process that occurs as a result of digesting and metabolising food.

Green tea is also one of the foods that may block angiogenesis (sorry, I have to slip one technical term in here). Angiogenesis refers to a process of blood vessel growth. For example, angiogenesis that builds up a blood supply to tumours can unfortunately make the tumours grow. Scientists have discovered that angiogenesis does the same thing with fat tissue: it creates a blood supply to fat tissue too, so it can grow. Fat tissue and cancer feed on oxygen delivered by these new blood vessels.

There's excellent science published in the best journals that something in green tea inhibits angiogenesis. The jury is still out on all this, but until we know more, I suggest drinking three cups of green tea a day.

Although doctors should set an example, I confess I'm not much of a green tea drinker. If I'm having a cup, I'm probably in an Asian restaurant. I promise to do better, though, and drink more green tea.

Coffee is also permitted on the 17 Day Diet. The caffeine kicks your metabolism into high gear. Caffeine also kick-starts the breakdown of fat in the body. One to two cups a day is ideal.

DOCTOR, CAN YOU PLEASE TELL ME ?

Am I allowed to I drink alcohol on the 17 Day Diet?

I knew you'd ask that. Alcohol can actually be good for you. Major studies have concluded that moderate alcohol consumption cuts heart attack risk in half, largely because drinkers have about 15 per cent higher levels of HDL cholesterol than non-drinkers, which prevents heart disease by cleansing the blood vessels of fatty build-ups. Moderate alcohol means one drink a day: 150 ml (5 fl oz) of wine, 350 ml (12 fl oz) of beer or 45 ml (1½ fl oz) of spirits.

Although a little alcohol is good for your heart, it's not that good for your waistline. Alcohol is dehydrating and interferes with fat-burning. The liver works overtime to metabolise the alcohol, so its job of burning fat gets less priority.

Once you get to Cycle 3, it's fine with me if you have one drink a day. Now, I don't recommend keeping it at your desk (at least not for daytime use), but I do recommend it, especially red wine. One of my hobbies outside of work is enjoying fine red wine. To pursue my passion for drinking and collecting fine red wine, I enjoy attending wine tastings with my friends.

Red wine contains resveratrol (a powerful antioxidant found in grape skin). It turns off a gene for certain inflammatory proteins. These proteins ride around in your bloodstream. When there's a foreign body, like a toxic molecule from an infection or a toxin, the proteins attach it to your arterial wall. This attachment stimulates inflammation. Inflammation can lead to clogged arteries, blood clots, impotence and even a heart attack or stroke. One glass of red wine a day may help prevent these things. So, cheers.

How Much Should You Weigh?

As you begin the 17 Day Diet, have a specific weight goal in mind. In other words aim for a weight at which you feel you will look your best. Keep in mind that there's really no such thing as the 'perfect' weight because we all come in a variety of body shapes, heights and bone structures. However, there are 'ideal weight ranges', so there is a simple equation I tend to follow:

If you're a woman: Start with 45.4 kg (100 lb) for the first 152.5 cm (5 ft) of your height, and add 2.5 kg (5 lb) for each extra 2.5 cm (1 in) to get the midpoint of what should be your ideal body weight range. Then you need to factor in your body structure. Some people are smaller boned; others are big boned. If you're small boned, subtract 15 per cent from the normal-framed weights; if you're large boned, add 15 per cent to the normal-framed weights. For a lot of people, that's too much maths. So I did the maths for you (in metric):

WOMEN		
Small-Boned Frame	**Midpoint**	**Large-Boned Frame**
152.5 cm = 38.5 kg	152.5 cm = 45.4 kg	152.5 cm = 52.2 kg
155 cm = 41 kg	155 cm = 47.6 kg	155 cm = 54.9 kg
157.5 cm = 42.6 kg	157.5 cm = 49.9 kg	157.5 cm = 57.6 kg
160 cm = 44.5 kg	160 cm = 52.2 kg	160 cm = 59.9 kg
162.5 cm = 46.3 kg	162.5 cm = 54.4 kg	162.5 cm = 62.1 kg
165 cm = 48 kg	165 cm = 56.7 kg	165 cm = 65.3 kg
167.5 cm = 49.9 kg	167.5 cm = 59 kg	167.5 cm = 68 kg
170 cm = 52.2 kg	170 cm = 61.2 kg	170 cm = 70.3 kg
172.5 cm = 54 kg	172.5 cm = 63.5 kg	172.5 cm = 73 kg
175 cm = 55.8 kg	175 cm = 65.8 kg	175 cm = 75.4 kg
177.5 cm = 58 kg	177.5 cm = 68 kg	177.5 cm = 78.5 kg
180 cm = 59.9 kg	180 cm = 70.8 kg	180 cm = 80.7 kg
182.5 cm = 61.7 kg	182.5 cm = 72.6 kg	182.5 cm = 83.5 kg

Need to convert from imperial? If you know your height in feet and inches, multiply the feet by 12 – remember from your old school days there are 12 inches to a foot – and add to the inches, then multiply that figure by 2.54 to get centimetres. So, if you are are 5 ft 4 in, 5 x 12 = 60 + 4 = 64, then 64 x 2.54 = 162.5 cm (or almost, 162.56 cm to be exact).

For weight, 1 pound = 0.4535 kilograms, so if you weigh 10 stone 3 lb (remember, 14 lb to a stone), 10 x 14 = 140 + 3 =143 lb; 143 x 0.4535 = 64.85 kg.

If you're a man: Take 49.9 kg (110 lb) for the first 152.5 cm (5 ft) of your height, and add 2.7 kg (6 lb) for each extra 2.5 cm (1 in) to get the midpoint of what should be your ideal body weight range. Allow for being small-boned or large-boned, as explained above.

MEN		
Small-Boned Frame	*Midpoint*	*Large-Boned Frame*
152.5 cm = 42.6 kg	152.5 cm = 49.9 kg	152.5 cm = 57.6 kg
155 cm = 44.9 kg	155 cm = 52.6 kg	155 cm = 60.3 kg
157.5 cm = 47.2 kg	157.5 cm = 55.3 kg	157.5 cm = 63.5 kg
160 cm = 49.4 kg	160 cm = 58 kg	160 cm = 66.7 kg
162.5 cm = 51.7 kg	162.5 cm = 60.8 kg	162.5 cm = 69.9 kg
165 cm = 54 kg	165 cm = 63.5 kg	165 cm = 73 kg
167.5 cm = 56.2 kg	167.5 cm = 66.2 kg	167.5 cm = 76.2 kg
170 cm = 58.5 kg	170 cm = 68.9 kg	170 cm = 79.4 kg
172.5 cm = 60.8 kg	172.5 cm = 71.7 kg	172.5 cm = 82.6 kg
175 cm = 63 kg	175 cm = 74.4 kg	175 cm = 85.7 kg
177.5 cm = 65.8 kg	177.5 cm = 77.1 kg	177.5 cm = 88.9 kg
180 cm = 68 kg	180 cm = 79.8 kg	180 cm = 91.6 kg
183 cm = 70.3 kg	183 cm = 82.6 kg	183 cm = 94.8 kg
185.5 cm = 72.6 kg	185.5 cm = 85.3 kg	185.5 cm = 98 kg
188 cm = 74.8 kg	188 cm = 88 kg	188 cm = 101.2 kg
190.5 cm = 77.1 kg	190.5 cm = 90.7 kg	190.5 cm = 104.3 kg
193 cm = 79.4 kg	193 cm = 93.4 kg	193 cm = 107.5 kg
195.5 cm = 81.4 kg	195.5 cm = 96.2 kg	195.5 cm = 110.7 kg
198 cm = 83.9 kg	198 cm = 98.9 kg	198 cm = 113.9 kg

How Often Should You Weigh Yourself?

Not too many people like to weigh themselves. Doctors know this. After patients step on the scales, they think they are giving them the weight of a completely different person, like Hulk Hogan. Since we don't weigh people naked, they tell us to subtract a few pounds for their shoes and jewellery. Some people strip off this stuff faster than lightning and step on the scales again. But doctors' scales

SCIENCE SAYS: Use Your Brain to Get Buff

Medical studies have shown that visualising yourself in the shape you want to be in can help you attain a trim, toned physique. The brain thinks very much in pictures. If you can call up a picture in your mind, you have a powerful way of making it happen. So it's important to get the image of your perfect body in your mind so you can create it.

Start imagining what your life will be like as a thin, healthy person. You'll be able to play, be active, really live and enjoy living for your family. You'll be able to shop at normal shops, not own plus-sized clothes and forget worrying about fitting into aeroplane seats. You'll no longer be a target of jokes or have people judge you. And you won't have to fear a future of diabetes, heart attack, stroke or other weight-related health issues. All of these images give your mind realistic goals to work towards.

do not lie. Patients have to accept the truth. Their bodies, without consulting them, have been converting muffins, pizza and ice cream into fat.

Let's talk about scales for a moment. Your bathroom scales can be a top tool for losing weight. I know, some people say throw them out. But those people are naturally thin or possibly teach aerobics classes. They don't need scales.

If you skirt the scales, your weight might start going up, and you won't know it. Then, when the nurse forces you at pen point to step on the scales at your next doctor's appointment and 136 kg (300 lb) pops up, you might go into shock.

Tracking your weight is one of the most important things you can do to prevent that happening. It's also a habit that has helped people in the National Weight Control Registry – a group in the US of 'successful losers' – hold their weight steady. Participants have lost at least 13.5 kg (30 lb) and kept it off for at least a year. Yes, other things can tell you a lot about your weight: the way your clothes fit, how winded you feel going up a flight of stairs or how you look in the mirror. But weigh yourself too, every few days, or at least once a week, and definitely after each 17 day Cycle. Just resist weighing yourself dozens of times a day in hopes of a better outcome.

So take that sweet tin off your desk. It may make you less popular with your co-workers, but you're on your way to a lighter life. And that's exciting.

LEAN 17: Facts about Fat

1. The average adult has 40 billion fat cells.

2. Fat is also one of the most abundant types of tissue in the body.

3. Fat tissue is a dynamic, complex and necessary component of life.

4. Girls are born with more fat cells than boys.

5. By the time you're a teenager, you are likely to have all the fat cells you are ever going to have.

6. Fat grows when existing cells enlarge and when new cells get created.

7. The number of fat cells can go up, but not down.

8. When you lose weight, existing fat cells shrink.

9. Fat cells die, but your body quickly replenishes them with the same number.

10. Fat cells are bigger in obese people.

11. Fat cells come in two types: white and brown. White is the kind that makes your jeans too tight. Brown fat is found in babies and has the ability to burn energy.

12. Fat cells, like cancer cells and other cells in the body, feed themselves oxygen with new blood vessels in a process known as angiogenesis. Fat can't expand without expanding its blood vessels, just like a city can't expand without expanding its roads. Researchers are studying whether certain cancer medicines can starve fat cells to stop fat expansion in the same way they starve tumours.

13. When you exercise, cells produce an enzyme that tells fatty tissue to release its stores for muscles to burn.

14. The liver stores glucose from food as glycogen and releases it into the bloodstream when energy is needed. Once glucose runs out, the body starts to burn fat.

15. Fat cells secrete oestrogen, which is linked to certain types of cancer, chiefly breast cancer in postmenopausal women.

16. Body fat accumulates from head to toe and comes off the same way.

17. Body fat is like a ski suit: it provides insulation against the cold. A downside of getting thin is that you might shiver more often.

Review:

- On the 17 Day Diet, you eat healthy foods: lean proteins, vegetables, low-sugar fruits, natural carbs, probiotics and friendly fats. These foods work together to improve your digestion and metabolism.

- The 17 Day Diet supplies the nutrients you need for good health.

- The 17 Day Diet limits carbs somewhat, because many people are carbohydrate sensitive, a condition that interferes with weight loss.

- Drinking water is vital for weight loss; so is drinking green tea.

3

Cycle 1: Accelerate

. . . .

Losing up to 4.5 or 5.4 kg (10 or 12 lb) over the next 17 days is possible, and you can see impressive results quickly if you follow to the letter Cycle 1: Accelerate.

The trouble with most diets (besides the boring food lists and the inevitable hunger pangs) is that it's tricky to find one that helps you shed weight quickly without compromising the nutritional quality of your meals – and ultimately your health and vitality. This Cycle gets you on the road to lean quickly, plus keeps you full, energetic and motivated.

On this Cycle you can eat unlimited protein – including meat, poultry, eggs and fish – as well as many vegetables. But you limit your carbohydrate intake by initially cutting out white bread, potatoes, pasta, rice, chocolate, biscuits and sugary puddings and sweets. Fruit and fats are not banned, and that's good because both will add sweetness and flavour to your diet.

Cycle 1 is called Accelerate because its purpose is to trigger rapid weight loss in a healthy manner by mobilising fat stores and flushing water and toxins from your system. The following are the things the Accelerate Cycle will be doing for you:

- Reducing carbohydrate intake so that your body taps into its storage fat.

- Increasing protein intake so that your body goes into a fat-burning mode.

- Correcting improper digestion – a situation that can hold you back from fat-burning.

- Providing rapid weight loss at the start, so that you have the incentive to keep going.

- Cutting out sugar, sweets, refined carbohydrates and other substances that cause those dreaded spikes and dips in blood sugar. Once you've broken the Cycle, your body will simply not crave them any more. In this Cycle you're removing foods that don't work well for your body.

- Clearing your body of possible toxins. Pollutants in the body interfere with both the thyroid gland, which helps regulate the body's metabolism, and individual cells' energy factories (mitochondria), which convert fuel into energy.

If you reach your goal after the first 17 days, you can go right on to Cycle 4, maintenance. If you still have more weight to lose, move on to Cycle 2: Activate – and enjoy even more foods for another 17 days. And then it's on to Cycle 3 for the next 17 days, a more liberal version of the first two Cycles. And if you're waiting for the day when I declare that cupcakes are part of your diet, that day arrives with Cycle 4, designed to keep your weight off with the reintroduction of your favourite foods back into your life.

SCIENCE SAYS: Toxins and Metabolic Rate

I wouldn't be surprised if our livers went around saying: 'I don't get no respect!' Day in and day out, we're exposed to toxins through drinking water, some foods and other sources. The liver, the primary organ of metabolism, has to work overtime to detoxify these things out of the body. Also, these particular toxins are stored in your fat cells – so as you start to lose weight, they're released into your bloodstream.

A team of Quebec researchers found that when toxins are released whilst overweight people are dieting, their metabolic rate – the speed at which calories are burnt – slows down considerably, even more than the slowdown often caused by dieting. Fortunately, many of the foods, particularly fruits and vegetables, on the 17 Day Diet are heroes at cleansing the body of toxins.

Source: *American Journal of Physiology—Regulatory, Integrative and Comparative Physiology, 2001.*

The Accelerate Cycle is the handiest diet tool you've got for getting – and keeping – your weight down. If your diet goes AWOL for whatever reason – and you gain some weight back, you can always return to the Accelerate Cycle to get back on track. Do this and you'll keep getting closer to your ideal weight. It's a short-term strategy that will guarantee long-term results.

My Hunger/Fullness Meter

Your parents probably drilled into you that you were not allowed to leave the table unless you finished everything on your plate. That was good advice when portions were smaller, and everyone hated to waste food.

These days, most of us don't know when we're hungry and when we're full. We lose this ability by the time we reach primary school. And it's making us fat.

I have a solution: Dr Mike's Hunger/Fullness Meter. The Fullness Meter is kind of like the 'pain scale' doctors ask you about when you are in the hospital. Basically, you rate your hunger and fullness on a scale. This is not a new idea; there are lots of hunger scales out there. But the problem with most is that they want you to rate your hunger on a scale of 0 to 10. That's too complicated. What is the difference between a 0 or a 1, or a 9 or a 10, anyway? You'll spend so much time trying to work out your rating that you won't have time to eat.

I say it's simpler to use a hunger rating from 1–2; and a fullness rating from 3–4. Here's how mine works.

Hunger Meter

1. **I'm little hungry; my stomach feels as hollow as the promises of a politician.**
   Eat now to prevent yourself from progressing to 2. Other leading indicators of mild hunger are slight stomach growling, mild headache, shakiness and loss of concentration. If you aren't sure whether you're actually hungry, you're probably not. You may be confusing true hunger with boredom, fatigue or thirst.

2. **I'm so hungry I could eat the lining of an empty Spam can. My stomach is growling so loud it scared off a stray dog. I've got to get something to eat, and fast.**
   Don't let yourself get here. You'll be frantically eating a sugar-laden cake or pie and downing a can of fizzy drink.

Fullness Meter

3. **I'm starting to feel full. I will stop now so that I can save on my food bill.**

   You have entered that pleasant zone where you are no longer hungry but not quite full either. Feel honourable about leaving a little room in your stomach. Try to keep yourself here at meals, never starving, never stuffed.

4. **I'm so stuffed I'll have to waddle over to the sofa to collapse.**

   You have eaten too much, even if it's all on your diet. Avoid this extreme; practise more restraint. Don't feel obliged to clear your plate, either. Stop eating as soon as your stomach feels full. Those extra bites of food that you're trying not to waste add unneeded calories.

As you go through your day and manage your mealtimes, ask yourself how hungry or full you are, based on my Hunger/Fullness Meter. Your goal is to listen to your body and let go of external cues such as the clock to tell you when and how much to eat.

General Guidelines for the Accelerate Cycle

1. Follow the Accelerate Cycle for 17 days. If you reach your weight loss goal, move on to Cycle 4: Arrive. If you have more weight to lose, go on to the next Cycle: Activate.

2. Your diet will consist of lean proteins, vegetables, low-sugar fruits, probiotic foods like yoghurt and good fats. Starchy foods such as potatoes, pulses, brown rice, corn and oats are not permitted on this Cycle.

3. Remove skin from chicken or turkey prior to cooking or purchase skinless poultry.

4. About eggs: You may eat up to two eggs a day. But stick to no more than four yolks per week if your doctor has diagnosed you with high cholesterol. Egg whites can be eaten without restriction.

5. Enjoy fresh vegetables and fruits as much as possible. For convenience frozen and canned items are fine, if chosen in moderation. They must be unsweetened, however.

6. Do not eat any fruit after 2.00 p.m. Fruit is a carb. The timing of carbohydrate intake is very important. I've found that carbs eaten early in the day supply the body with only enough fuel (in the form of glycogen

stored in muscles) to energise the body the rest of the day. You'll find that this approach also improves your waistline. If you eat carbs in the evening, it's harder for the body to burn them off because you expend less energy in the evening. Those carbs might be stored as fat.

7. Avoid alcohol and sugar in order to help your body eliminate toxins, improve digestion and burn fat.

8. Adopt the habit of drinking green tea. It contains some caffeine but offers compounds that help burn fat.

9. Research indicates that probiotic foods boost the immune system and promote intestinal-cleansing bacteria. Probiotic foods are also thought to help the body burn fat. If you don't like yoghurt, try sugar-free fruit-flavoured yoghurt or cultured milk, such as low-fat acidophilus milk (it tastes just like regular semi-skimmed milk). Also, you can still get the friendly bacteria you need. Most health food shops sell capsules containing probiotics; follow the manufacturer's instructions for dosage.

10. Eat slowly and only until full; do not overload your stomach.

11. Drink eight 240 ml (8 fl oz) glasses of pure water a day.

12. Exercise at least 17 minutes a day.

Take It Off: The Accelerate Cycle Food List

Lean Proteins

Here's where you'll be getting a lot of your fat-burning power. Eat all you want of the following proteins. They're freebies. The 17 Day Diet is purposely high in protein because it stimulates the reduction of body fat.

Fish*

Salmon, canned or fresh

Sole

Plaice

Red snapper

Tilapia

Canned light tuna (in water)

*Opt for wild-caught rather than farm-raised fish, which may have received doses of antibiotics. Avoid the bigger fish such as swordfish, shark, king mackerel and albacore tuna. They are the most likely to carry metals such as methyl-mercury, which is considered a toxin.

Poultry

Chicken breasts
Turkey breasts
Turkey mince, lean
Eggs (2 eggs = 1 serving)
Egg whites (4 egg whites = 1 serving)

Cleansing Vegetables

Eat all you want from the following list. They're freebies too. I call these cleansing vegetables because they support detoxification in the intestines, blood and liver, and offer protective antioxidants. A few honourable mentions:

Cauliflower, cabbage, broccoli and Brussels sprouts supply important phytochemicals (disease-fighting substances in plants), which help the liver detoxify chemicals, medicines and pollutants.

Asparagus, spinach and okra are all notable sources of glutathione, a vital compound that aids in the removal of fat-soluble toxins. (So is cooked chicken.)

Spinach, broccoli, tomatoes and Brussels sprouts contribute alpha-lipoic acid, a powerful antioxidant that destroys harmful free radicals, which are by-products of detoxification.

Onions accelerate the break down of fats in your food. As a result your body is more apt to excrete them than to store them in fat cells.

Salad leaves have diuretic properties (which help you lose water weight), and their ability to stabilise blood sugar prevents binge eating.

Globe artichokes have a range of health-promoting benefits. This veggie scores high on the antioxidant scale, thanks to the presence of cynarin and silymarin. These two phytochemicals are thought to lower cholesterol, protect liver cells from toxins, enhance circulation, alpha-lipoic acid and aid digestion. Both antioxidants are found in the leaves and the heart of the vegetable.

Asparagus	Carrots
Aubergine	Cauliflower
Broccoli	Celery
Brussels sprouts	Cucumbers
Cabbage	French beans

LEAN 17: Maximise the Health Power of Fruits and Veggies

1. Look for fresh produce that is crisp and not wilted. Fresh = nutritious.

2. When buying fresh fruits, look for bruises. Bruising initiates a chemical reaction that saps the nutrient content.

3. When purchasing pre-packed salads, look for a colourful medley of greens in the packet. The more colour, the more antioxidants and phytochemicals in the vegetables.

4. Always select the brightest, most colourful fruits and vegetables on the shelves. The brighter the colour, the more vitamins and nutrients in the produce.

5. Go for darker shades of green when buying lettuces. Dark-leafed lettuces such as cos are richer in certain B vitamins than lighter varieties of lettuce such as iceberg.

6. Buy vegetables such as onions and peppers in all their various colours for a greater array of nutrients.

7. Purchase fresh fruits and vegetables in season when their flavour and nutrition are at peak levels.

8. Buy locally grown fruits and vegetables when you can. They tend to be more nutrient-rich because they come picked straight from the field. (A lot of nutrient loss occurs when produce is in transit for delivery to supermarkets.)

9. Berries are highly perishable. At the supermarket look at the base of the container. Staining is a sign that the fruit has been bruised or is overripe. Nutrient loss has already set in, and the fruit will spoil rapidly.

10. Look for the brightest strawberries possible. A bright colour signals exceptional nutrient quality. If berries show too much whiteness at their base, they're less nutritious.

11. Sniff berries to test for freshness. A pleasant aroma indicates good flavour, ripeness and nutritional goodness.

12. Buy a variety of fruits and vegetables on the food lists. The greater the variety of foods you eat, the healthier your nutrition.

13. Eat fruits and vegetables raw whenever possible. Generally, raw produce is healthier. Exceptions to the raw rule: cooked carrots and tomatoes yield more antioxidants.

continued on the next page

14. Cook vegetables the shortest time possible to preserve nutrients.

15. Steaming vegetables is a great way to keep nutrients from escaping.

16. Avoid thawing frozen fruits and vegetables prior to cooking. As foods thaw, micro-organisms possibly present in food may begin to multiply, spoiling the food.

17. In most cases avoid peeling. Nutrients and fibre are lost when produce is peeled.

Garlic	Mushrooms
Green, leafy vegetables	Okra
(including beetroot greens,	Onions
turnip greens, spring greens)	Parsley
Globe artichoke	Peppers, green, orange, red, yellow
Globe artichoke hearts	Spinach
Kale	Spring onions
Leeks	Tomatoes
Lettuces, all varieties	Watercress

Low-Sugar Fruit – 2 servings daily

Low-sugar fruits are good sources of fibre that provide bulk and digest slowly, helping you feel full. They're also full of water, high in fibre and super low in calories, which makes them ideal for weight loss.

Apples	Pears
Berries, all types	Plums
Grapefruit	Prickly pear cactus
Oranges	Prunes
Peaches	Red grapes

Probiotic Foods – 2 servings daily

Probiotics help balance your digestive system, resulting in an overall increase in the efficiency of digestion. Research shows that probiotics may also help fight obesity. If you've been under stress, taken antibiotics or eaten a lot of foods packaged with preservatives, these things can kill off the beneficial bugs in your system – so eating more probiotic foods is a good idea.

DOCTOR, CAN YOU PLEASE TELL ME

What if I take a medicine that interacts with grapefruit?

Grapefruit and grapefruit juice (which you do not drink on the 17 Day Diet) interacts with a few specific prescription drugs, and one is statins, taken to lower cholesterol. Grapefruit and grapefruit juice may prevent the liver from sufficiently breaking down the drug, resulting in a higher dose entering the bloodstream. Most doctors know this.

This interaction was discovered back in the 1990s with research studies. A handful of these studies talked about the "usual dose" of grapefruit juice. But the usual dose was sometimes a whole quart a day! No one drinks that much grapefruit juice, even if grapefruit juice is your favorite food.

Personally, I like grapefruit. I eat it for its taste, vitamin C and fiber. Plus, I like folding the grapefruit in half and squeezing the juice into a spoon.

What I tell my patients who take statins is that they may enjoy half a grapefruit or 240 ml/8 fl oz of grapefruit juice (no juice on the Accelerate Cycle of the 17 Day Diet, though) in the morning.

Secondly, I instruct them to always take their statins in the evening. These measures help minimise any grapefruit-drug interaction. And they still get to squeeze their grapefruit.

Before doing these things, you should be sure to consult with your own GP.

There's no recommendation for probiotics. To maintain health, a probiotic count of 5 to 10 billion is adequate. That may sound like a lot, but consider this: a 175 g (6 oz) serving of yoghurt contains around 17 billion probiotics.

Yoghurt, any type, including Greek-style, sugar-free fruit-flavoured, natural and low-fat (175 g/6 oz = 1 serving)

Kefir: similar to a drinking-style yoghurt; great for making smoothies (240 ml/8 fl oz = 1 serving)

Yakult (small 50-calorie bottle)

Probiotic cottage cheese (115 g/4 oz = 1 serving)

Reduced salt miso dissolved in low-fat, low-sodium broth (1 tablespoon = 1 serving)

Tempeh, a fermented cake of pressed soya beans (115 g/4 oz = I serving)

Sauerkraut (115 g/4 oz = 1 serving)

Kimchi, a Korean cabbage (45 g/1½oz = 1 serving) – find it in Asian supermarkets, and enjoy a small amount as a side dish with meals.

Friendly Fats: 1 to 2 tablespoons daily

I don't purposely tell my patients to eat fats, unless it's the healthy kind such as fish oil, olive oil or linseed (flaxseed) oil. These healthful fats can help reduce the risk of heart disease, stroke, certain cancers and diabetes, as well as promote joint health, prevent muscle loss and encourage fat loss and muscle toning.

Olive oil

Linseed oil

Condiments

Condiments and seasonings are allowed in moderation: salsa, low-carb pasta sauce, light soy sauce, low-cal tomato ketchup, fat-free sour cream, low-fat, low-sodium broth, sugar-free jams and jellies, vegetable oil cooking spray, fat-free cheeses (i.e. Parmesan), fat-free salad dressing, salt, pepper, vinegar, mustard, herbs and spices.

Meal Planning Made Easy

It's easy to remember what to eat during this Cycle:

- As much as you want of specific proteins and cleansing vegetables.
- Supplement these foods with 2 low-sugar fruits daily; 2 servings of probiotic foods such as yoghurt, kefir, Yakult (small 50-calorie bottle), reduced salt miso dissolved in low-fat, low-sodium broth, sauerkraut (115 g/4 oz a serving) and 1 to 2 tablespoons of friendly fat. It's that easy.

You do not have to count anything, except your 2 daily fruit servings, your 2 daily probiotic servings and your fat serving.

Here is a typical day on the Accelerate Cycle:

Breakfast

- 2 eggs or 4 egg whites, prepared without oil; or 1 serving probiotic food such as yoghurt
- 1 fruit serving
- 1 cup green tea

DOCTOR, CAN YOU PLEASE TELL ME

Can I take a probiotic supplement instead of eating probiotic foods?

Yes. Probiotics come in supplement form that you can buy at your pharmacy or health food shop. Look for a probiotic supplement that contains 10 to 20 billion colony-forming units (CFUs), and read the label to learn how it should be stored.

Lunch

* Liberal amounts of protein in the form of fish, poultry or eggs plus unlimited amounts of cleansing vegetables; or 1 probiotic serving plus unlimited amounts of cleansing vegetables
* 1 cup green tea

Dinner

* Liberal amounts of protein in the form of fish or chicken
* Unlimited amounts of cleansing vegetables
* 1 cup green tea

Snacks

* 2nd fruit serving
* 2nd probiotic serving

Additional

* 1 serving (1 to 2 tablespoons) of friendly fat to use on salads, vegetables or for cooking

17 Sample Menus

Here are examples of how you can create your daily menu during the Accelerate Cycle. You may follow these exactly or create your own menus based on the above guidelines. Some days include easy-to-make recipes, shown in italics. You'll find these in the Appendix.

Wake-up drink

Every morning, as soon as you rise, drink one 240 ml (8 fl oz) cup of hot water. Squeeze half a lemon into the cup; the lemon stimulates your digestive juices. Your goal is to drink at least seven more glasses of water by the end of the day.

The rate at which you burn calories drops if you're dehydrated. And if you're dehydrated, your body doesn't absorb nutrients properly. 'Negative waters' such as coffee or tea do not count towards your total daily fluid intake.

First consult your doctor regarding the amount of your daily water intake if you have been diagnosed with congestive heart failure. Water requirements vary.

Day 1

Breakfast
* 2 scrambled egg whites
* ½ grapefruit, or other fresh fruit
* 1 cup of green tea

Lunch
* Large green salad topped with tuna; drizzle with 1 tablespoon of olive or linseed oil and 2 tablespoons balsamic vinegar
* 1 cup green tea

Dinner
* Plenty of grilled chicken with liberal amounts of any vegetables from the list, steamed or raw
* 1 cup green tea

Snacks
* 175 g/6 oz of sugar-free natural yoghurt or other probiotic serving mixed with 1 to 2 tablespoons sugar-free jam
* 1 serving of fruit from the list

Day 2

Breakfast

* 175 g/6 oz natural low-fat yoghurt, mixed with 115 g/4 oz berries or other fruit (chopped) on the list. You may sweeten the mixture with 1 packet of natural low-calorie sweetener or sugar-free fruit jam
* 1 cup green tea

Lunch

* *Super Salad* (large salad with a generous bed of salad leaves and salad vegetables of your choice – tomatoes, onions, cucumbers, celery, etc. – drizzled with 1 tablespoon of olive oil or linseed oil and 2 tablespoons herbed vinegar or vinegar of your choice)
* 1 cup green tea

Dinner

* Plenty of grilled or baked salmon with liberal amounts of any vegetables from the list, steamed or raw
* 1 cup green tea

Snacks

* 175 g/6 oz sugar-free fruit-flavoured yoghurt or 1 cup natural low-fat yoghurt, sweetened with a natural low-calorie sweetener or a table-spoon of sugar-free fruit jam
* 1 serving of fruit

Day 3

Breakfast

* 2 hard-boiled or poached eggs
* ½ grapefruit or other fresh fruit in season
* 1 cup green tea

Lunch

* 1 large bowl of *Chicken-Vegetable Soup*
* 1 cup green tea

Dinner

* Plenty of roast turkey breast or turkey fillets, steamed carrots and steamed asparagus
* 1 cup green tea

Snacks

* 175 g/6 oz natural low-fat yoghurt, sweetened with a natural low-calorie sweetener or a tablespoon of sugar-free fruit jam
* *Kefir Smoothie:* Mix 240 ml (8 fl oz) of kefir with 115 g/4 oz of frozen unsweetened berries, sugar-free fruit jam and 1 tablespoon linseed oil. Blend until smooth

Day 4

Breakfast

* *Kefir Smoothie*
* 1 cup green tea

Lunch

* *Marinated Vegetable Salad* or *Super Salad*
* 175 g/6 oz natural low-fat yoghurt with a sliced fresh peach, or other fruit in season, for dessert
* 1 cup green tea

Dinner

* *Aubergine Parmesan*
* Alternative dinner: Any of the lean proteins with plenty of cooked cleansing vegetables from the list
* 1 cup green tea

Day 5

Breakfast

* 2 scrambled egg whites
* ½ grapefruit or other fresh fruit in season
* 1 cup green tea

Lunch

* Salad of baby spinach leaves, cherry tomatoes and crumbled low-fat feta or blue cheese; drizzle with 1 tablespoon of olive or linseed oil and 2 tablespoons balsamic vinegar
* 1 cup green tea

Dinner

* Turkey burgers, with side salad drizzled with 1 tablespoon of olive or linseed oil and 2 tablespoons balsamic vinegar
* 1 cup green tea

Snacks

* 115 g/4 oz of fresh berries
* 175 g/6 oz natural low-fat yoghurt, sweetened with natural low-calorie sweetener or a tablespoon of sugar-free fruit jam

Day 6

Breakfast

* 175 g/6 oz natural low-fat yoghurt, mixed with 115 g/4 oz berries or other fruit (chopped) on the list. You may sweeten the mixture with 1 packet of natural low-calorie sweetener or a tablespoon of sugar-free fruit jam
* 1 cup green tea

Lunch

* *Lettuce Wraps* or grilled chicken breast with tossed salad drizzled with 1 tablespoon of olive or linseed oil and 2 tablespoons balsamic vinegar
* 1 cup green tea

Dinner

* *Sesame Fish*, or any grilled or baked fish
* Steamed cleansing vegetables
* 1 cup green tea

Snacks

* 2nd fruit serving of your choice
* 2nd probiotic serving of your choice

Day 7

Breakfast

* 2 scrambled eggs, 4 scrambled egg whites or 1 scrambled egg plus 2 scrambled egg whites. Top with salsa (optional)
* 1 apple or 115 g/4 oz fresh berries
* 1 cup green tea

Lunch
* *Taco Salad*
* 1 cup green tea

Dinner
* A stir-fry of vegetables (broccoli, onions, julienne carrots, red pepper, etc.), and chicken strips with 1 tablespoon of olive oil. Season with a little garlic, ginger and light soy sauce.
* 1 cup green tea

Snacks
* 2nd fruit serving plus 1 probiotic serving of your choice
* 2nd probiotic serving of your choice

Day 8

Breakfast
* 175 g/6 oz natural low-fat yoghurt, mixed with 115 g/4 oz berries or other fruit (chopped) on the list. You may sweeten the mixture with 1 packet of natural low-calorie sweetener or a tablespoon of sugar-free fruit jam.
* 1 cup green tea

Lunch
* Salmon salad: 2 large handfuls of salad vegetables (lettuce, tomatoes, onions, cucumbers, etc.), baked or canned salmon, drizzled with 1 tablespoon olive or linseed oil, mixed with 2 tablespoons balsamic vinegar and seasonings.
* 1 cup green tea

Dinner
* Turkey burgers (made with lean turkey mince)
* Steamed vegetables (choose from list of cleansing vegetables)
* Side salad drizzled with 1 tablespoon olive or linseed oil, mixed with 2 tablespoons balsamic vinegar and seasonings
* 1 cup green tea

Snacks
* 2nd fruit serving
* 2nd probiotic serving

Day 9

Breakfast
- *Greek Egg Scramble*
- 1 fresh orange
- 1 cup green tea

Lunch
- *Salad Niçoise*
- 1 cup green tea

Dinner
- Grilled chicken breast (marinate in fat-free Italian dressing, then broil or grill)
- Steamed vegetables (choose from list of cleansing vegetables)
- 1 cup green tea

Snacks
- *Kefir Smoothie*
- 2nd probiotic serving

Day 10

Breakfast
115 g/4 oz cottage cheese
1 medium pear, sliced
1 cup green tea

Lunch
Balsamic Artichoke (use fat-free salad dressing as a dipping sauce)
1 medium apple
1 cup green tea

Dinner
- *Oven Barbecued Chicken Breast*
- Side salad drizzled with 1 tablespoon olive or linseed oil, mixed with 2 tablespoons balsamic vinegar and seasonings
- 1 cup green tea

Snacks
- 2nd probiotic serving
- Raw, cut-up veggies

Day 11

Breakfast
- Yoghurt Smoothie: 120 ml (4 fl oz) kefir, 85 g (3 oz) sugar-free fruit-flavoured yoghurt, and 115 g/4 oz berries (mix together in a blender)
- 1 cup green tea

Lunch
- *Super Salad*
- 1 cup green tea

Dinner
- *Turkey Black Bean Chilli*
- Side salad drizzled with 1 tablespoon olive or linseed oil, mixed with 2 tablespoons balsamic vinegar and seasonings
- 1 cup green tea

Snacks
- 2 probiotic servings

Day 12

Breakfast
- 2 hard-boiled or poached eggs
- ½ grapefruit or other fresh fruit in season
- 1 cup green tea

Lunch
- Baked or grilled chicken breast
- Tomatoes, sliced or stewed
- 1 medium orange
- 1 cup green tea

Dinner
- Baked or grilled fish, any kind from the list
- Cleansing vegetables, as many from the list as you wish
- 1 cup green tea

Snacks
- *Kefir Smoothie:* Mix 240 ml (8 fl oz) kefir with 115 g/4 oz of berries, sugar-free fruit jam and 1 tablespoon linseed oil and blend until smooth.
- 2nd probiotic serving

Day 13

Breakfast
* *Kefir Smoothie*
* 1 cup green tea

Lunch
* Tuna tossed with 1 tablespoon olive oil and a tablespoon of vinegar, served over a generous bed of lettuce
* 1 cup green tea

Dinner
* Plenty of roast turkey or chicken
* Tomato and onion salad, tossed with fat-free salad dressing
* 1 cup green tea

Snacks
* 2nd fruit serving
* 2nd probiotic serving

Day 14

Breakfast
* 2 scrambled eggs, 4 scrambled egg whites, or 1 scrambled egg plus 2 scrambled egg whites. Top with salsa (optional)
* 1 apple or 115 g/4 oz fresh berries
* 1 cup green tea

Lunch
* 1 large bowl of *Chicken-Vegetable Soup*
* 1 cup green tea

Dinner
* Plenty of grilled chicken or fish
* Generous portion of mixed steamed vegetables
* 1 cup green tea

Snacks
* 1 medium pear or other fruit in season
* 2nd probiotic serving of your choice

Day 15

Breakfast
- 115 g/4 oz cottage cheese
- 1 medium pear, sliced
- 1 cup green tea

Lunch
- *Aubergine Parmesan*
- 1 cup green tea

Dinner
- Plenty of browned lean turkey mince
- *Marinated Vegetable Salad*
- 1 cup green tea

Snacks
- 2nd fruit serving of your choice
- 2nd probiotic serving of your choice

Day 16

Breakfast
- *Spanish Omelette*
- ½ grapefruit or 1 medium orange
- 1 cup green tea

Lunch
- *Spicy Yoghurt Dip and Veggies*
- 1 cup green tea

Dinner
- Plenty of roast turkey breast or turkey fillets, steamed carrots and steamed asparagus
- 1 cup green tea

Snacks
- 2nd fruit serving
- 175 g/6 oz yoghurt

Day 17

Breakfast

- Smoothie: 240 ml (8 fl oz) kefir and 115 g/4 oz berries (mix together in a blender)
- 1 cup green tea

Lunch

- *Super Salad*
- 1 cup green tea

Dinner

- Steamed plaice or sole with lemon pepper
- Steamed broccoli
- 1 cup green tea

Snacks

- 1 medium apple or other fruit in season
- 2nd probiotic serving of your choice

Accelerate Cycle Worksheet

It may help you to plan your meals using the following worksheet. Using the food lists, simply fill in what you will eat each day.

Breakfast

Protein or probiotic serving: _____

Fruit serving: _____

Lunch

Protein or probiotic serving: _____

Cleansing vegetables: _____

Dinner

Protein serving: _____

Cleansing vegetables: _____

Snacks

2nd fruit serving: _____

2nd probiotic serving: _____

Other

Friendly fat serving: _____

Your eating habits may be a lot closer to horrible than healthy right now. That means it's time to hand out notices to muffins, pizzas, burgers, shakes and chips. Your stomach is about to welcome some healthier inhabitants, and I'm going to help you understand what it's like to feel good, and understand the connection between the choices you make and how you feel. For the first 17 days that you follow this diet, you will experience an entirely new energy, and you will see how quickly it can happen and how much better you can feel.

See you (hopefully less of you) in 17 days!

Review

- Cycle 1: Accelerate – kick-starts your weight loss.
- This Cycle reduces carb intake and increases protein intake.
- This Cycle clears your body of sugars and toxins to pave the way for weight loss.
- Use my Hunger/Fullness Meter to help you eat just the right amount of food for your body.
- Use this Cycle as a tool to re-ignite weight loss if you ever have a slip and need to get back on track.

THE 17 MINUTE WORKOUT: Get in Two Quickies

Not those kinds of quickies (although you burn calories that way too). What I had in mind are two mini aerobic workouts: 17 minutes in the morning, and 17 minutes in the afternoon or early evening. Science already tells us that exercise boosts your metabolism for a few hours afterwards, so just think: you'll nearly double the afterburn if you split it up. Aerobic exercise includes fast walking, jogging, running, exercising on cardio machines and anything that gets your heart pumping for 17 minutes.

The Fibre Factor

E veryone knows about fibre. It is the indigestible part of plant foods our body cannot use for energy. Fibre, which sometimes used to be referred to as 'roughage', travels through our digestive tract creating bulky, soft stools that pass easily. Without adequate fibre, things get stopped up.

The 17 Day Diet is high in fibre on purpose. A growing body of research shows that high-fibre eating helps peel off pounds and banish them for good. Fibre does this mainly by curtailing your food intake. Specifically, fibrous foods provide bulk and stimulate the release of appetite-suppressing hormones. As a result you feel full whilst eating a meal, so you're less tempted to overeat.

High-fibre foods also take longer to chew. You may have to chew some foods 42 times before swallowing them. High-fibre foods may even have negative calories, because by the time you have finished chewing them, you have burnt up more calories than the food provides. Chewing also makes your meals last longer. That's nice, since it takes about 20 minutes after starting a meal for your body to send signals that it's full. And, when eaten with other nutrients, fibre slows the rate of digestion too, curbing your appetite between meals.

Eating more fibre-rich foods will have your body running strangely. So make sure you have a good book and some nice soft toilet paper to hand. All of this is good for weight loss, though. The fibre accelerates the time it takes for food to move through your intestinal tract. This means fewer calories are left to be stored as fat.

Attention, everyone reading this: if you eat too much food with a lot of fibre and don't drink enough water, you will have to buy a laxative. Fibre needs water to move through your system, or it will harden up like a block of cement in your colon.

4

Cycle 2:
Activate

· · · · · · · · · · · · ·

If **you've been** on other diets, you're all too aware of the standard outcome: You cut back on your food and you lose weight ... at least initially.
But then your progress slows to a crawl, before lagging or sometimes stopping altogether. Your body's natural tendency to preserve itself and its fat, at
all costs, kicks in. The Activate Cycle corrects this, resetting your metabolism,
so that your body stays in a fat-burning mode.

This Cycle is easy to follow too: You alternate your Cycle 1: Accelerate days
with Cycle 2: Activate days. In other words, you use this Cycle by spending
one day on the Activate diet and the next on the Accelerate diet, switching
between the two, one day at a time, as you progress towards your goal weight
over the next 17 days. Another way to look at it: on odd days you follow the
Activate Cycle; on even days, the Accelerate Cycle.

The approach of alternating Accelerate days with Activate days is based
on the scientifically validated mechanism of 'alternate-day fasting' (although
there is no fasting on this diet in the true sense of the word). In a nutshell
this means alternating low-calorie days with higher-calorie days in order to
lose body fat. Scientists at the University of California have led the way in
this cutting-edge research, with both human and rat studies. (How many of
these furry creatures have lost weight in order to save humanity from obesity
during the past 50 years is a mystery to me.)

Publishing much of their research in recent issues of the *American Journal of Clinical Nutrition*, these scientists have unearthed intriguing findings. Alternate-day fasting can:

* Trigger sustained weight loss (no frustrating plateaus). The weight that is lost is mostly fat.

* Activate the 'skinny' gene, which tells cells to burn – rather than hold on to – fat.

* Reduce the risk of heart disease by lowering levels of bad cholesterol and triglycerides, decreasing blood pressure and lowering heart rate.

* Alternating your food intake is a powerful concept in weight management. Here's a look at what this will be doing for you:

* Stripping away body fat. Your carb intake is still relatively low on this Cycle. When you cut carbs, your muscles give up stored carbohydrates, called muscle glycogen, as energy. In general when glycogen levels fall, the body increases its ability to burn body fat, so it makes sense to reduce your carbohydrate intake. When that happens the body increases fat burning.

* Giving momentum to your metabolism. This potent diet strategy seems to keep the metabolism elevated. It keeps your body guessing, as opposed to letting it get accustomed to one particular way of eating day after day. Just as you need to change things up in workouts for continued progress to avoid plateaus, you mustn't let your body get too comfortable with the foods you eat. It's all about shocking the metabolism to elicit a positive response.

* Taming your appetite. On the Activate Cycle, you get to eat some starchy carbs. But not just any carbs. You'll eat natural, slow-digesting carbs such as oats, wholegrains, brown rice, beans and pulses and sweet potatoes – a whole slew of carbs. Slow carbs take a longer time to reach the blood, which helps you feel full.

* Preventing carb sensitivity. Carbs are beneficial in that they help set up the body hormonally for muscle-toning if you exercise. They spark the release of insulin, which gets protein and carbs into muscles for growth and repair. The downside is that when you take in too many carbs, they can be readily converted to body fat and stored. On the Activate Cycle,

you're limited to no more than two servings of slow, natural carbs a day. This is the amount most people – especially women – are physiologically capable of tolerating in order to sustain fat metabolism.

Another major difference between the two Cycles is that you get to enjoy a greater variety of lean proteins, including shellfish and beef.

DOCTOR, CAN YOU PLEASE TELL ME ?

Wouldn't it just be easier to prescribe diet pills for weight loss?

Pharmaceutical companies are always racing to develop new weight-loss medicines, but they haven't had much luck. Even in the US, only three medicines have been approved in the past 30 years for treating obesity, one of which was withdrawn for safety reasons. I don't know what they did with the leftover tablets. Maybe they were recycled into something a dieter could use such as exercise bands.

The medicines that remain – orlistat and sibutramine – have been moderately successful. But I'm not an advocate of taking tablets for every little thing. Tablets don't fully address the problem. By prescribing medicines instead of lifestyle changes, doctors ignore the unhealthy habits that have contributed to obesity. One of these diet tablets, the 'fat blocker' orlistat, must be accompanied by a low-calorie diet to reduce your weight by about 5 per cent for most. Diets are vital, pills or no pills.

There's an 'yuck' factor with this particular medicine. Fat isn't absorbed, so it has to go somewhere. And orlistat takers find out in a hurry just where. (Keep an extra pair of underwear with you, or wear a nappy.)

But yes, some people's obesity is so out of control that it might be dangerous, and I might prescribe one of these medicines.

About the only advice doctors can give is stop eating sweets, fat, butter, puddings, super-burgers – basically, we want you to avoid anything the least bit tasty. We would make everyone do this if we could. Then we could stop worrying about the obesity epidemic and get back to other things like curing the common cold and filling out red tape.

General Guidelines for the Activate Cycle

1. Stay on the Activate Cycle for 17 days. The Activate Cycle consists of alternating between Activate days and Accelerate days.

2. Remove skin from chicken or turkey prior to cooking or purchase skinless poultry.

3. Trim all visible fat from meat.

4. About eggs: you may eat up to two eggs a day. But have no more than four yolks per week if your doctor has diagnosed you with high cholesterol. Egg whites can be eaten without restriction.

5. Keep gobbling up those fresh fruits and vegetables before they become worthy of a science experiment in the vegetable bin. For convenience frozen and tinned items are fine, if chosen in moderation. These products should be unsweetened, however.

6. Continue to avoid alcohol and sugar in order to help your body eliminate toxins, improve digestion and burn fat.

7. Don't eat more than two servings daily from the natural starches list.

8. Do not eat your fruit or natural starch serving past 2.00 p.m.

SCIENCE SAYS: Just a Single High-Fat Meal Does Heart Damage

Eating just one single high-fat meal makes your blood pressure go sky high, according to a study by US and Canadian researchers. They fed 30 healthy people a single meal that was either very low-fat (1% of calories) or very high-fat (46% of calories). The high-fat meal was a McDonald's breakfast; the healthier low-fat meal was cereal and low-fat yoghurt. The people were then exposed to stressful situations such as public speaking, performing mental maths and exposure to cold temperatures. Compared to the people given the low-fat meal, those who ate the high-fat meal experienced a greater jump in blood pressure and more stress on their blood vessels. These effects may cause harm to cardiovascular health. So much for the adage, 'All things in moderation'.

Source: *Journal of Nutrition*, April 2007.

9. Eat slowly and only until full; do not overload your stomach. Use my Hunger/Fullness Meter.

10. Drink eight 240 ml (8 fl oz) glasses of pure water a day.

11. Exercise for at least 17 minutes a day.

Take More Off: The Activate Cycle Food List

On the Activate Cycle, you'll be adding new foods to those you ate on the Accelerate Cycle. These additional foods are listed below.

Proteins

Add in the following foods:

Shellfish:

Clams   Crab   Mussels   Oysters   Scallops   Prawns

Lean Cuts of Meat* (The leanest cuts are those from the part of the animal that gets the most exercise. Therefore, cuts from the topside, silverside, chuck, and flank are the best.)

Beef topside	Pork boneless roast
Braising steak	Pork chops
Lean steak mince	Pork fillet
Rump steak	Lamb shoulder
Sirloin beef	Leg of lamb
Skirt steak	Veal cutlet

*Lean cuts tend to be a little tougher. You can tenderise lean cuts by marinating in fat-free liquids such as fruit juice, wine, fat-free salad dressings or fat-free broth.

Natural Starches

Grains: (1 serving)

Amaranth (100 g/3½ oz)	Basmati rice (100 g/3½ oz)
Barley, pearl (100 g/3½ oz)	Brown rice (100 g/3½ oz)

Bulgar wheat (70 g/2½ oz)

Couscous (100 g/3½ oz)

Millet (100 g/3½ oz)

Oat bran (45 g/1½ oz)

Polenta/cornmeal (70 g/2½ oz)

Porridge oats (45 g/1½ oz)

Quinoa (70 g/2½ oz)

Pulses: (1 serving)

Black beans (100 g/3½ oz)

Black-eyed beans (100 g/3½ oz)

Butter beans (100 g/3½ oz)

Chickpeas (125 g/4½ oz)

Kidney beans (100 g/3½ oz)

Lentils (100 g/3½ oz)

Haricot beans (100 g/3½ oz)

Peas (70 g/2½ oz)

Pinto bean (100 g/3½ oz)

Soya beans (100 g/3½ oz)

Split peas (100 g/3½ oz)

Starchy Vegetables: (1 serving)

Potato *(1 medium)*

Sweetcorn (70 g/2½ oz))

Sweet potato *(1 medium)*

Taro, available in Caribbean grocers *(1 serving = 55 g/2 oz)*

Winter squashes, acorn, butter-nut, etc. *(65 g/2¼ oz)*

Yam *(1 medium)*

Cleansing Vegetables
(Same foods as Accelerate Cycle)

Low-Sugar Fruits
(Same foods as Accelerate Cycle)

Probiotics
(Same foods as Accelerate cycle)

Friendly Fats
(Same foods as Accelerate cycle)

Condiments
Condiments and seasonings are allowed in moderation: salsa, low-carb pasta sauce, light soy sauce, low-cal tomato ketchup, fat-free sour

cream, low-fat, low-sodium broth, a natural low-calorie sweetener, sugar-free jams and jellies, vegetable oil cooking spray, fat-free cheeses (i.e. Parmesan), fat-free salad dressing, salt, pepper, vinegar, mustard, herbs and spices.

Meal Planning Made Easy

On Activate days, you eat:

* Liberal amounts of protein and cleansing vegetables
* Two daily servings of natural starches (carbohydrates)
* Two low-sugar fruit servings
* Two servings of probiotic foods
* One daily serving of friendly fat

Here's a typical day on the Activate Cycle:

Breakfast
* about 45 g/1½ oz hot wholegrain cereal or 2 eggs or 4 egg whites, prepared without oil; 1 *Dr Mike's Power Cookie*; or one probiotic serving
* 1 fruit serving
* 1 cup green tea

Lunch
* Liberal amounts of protein in the form of fish, shellfish, meat or chicken or eggs; or vegetables plus 1 probiotic serving
* 1 serving natural starch
* Unlimited amounts of cleansing vegetables
* 1 cup green tea

Dinner
* Liberal amounts of protein in the form of fish, shellfish, meat, or chicken or turkey
* Unlimited amounts of cleansing vegetables
* 1 cup green tea

Snacks
* 2nd fruit serving
* 2nd probiotic serving

Additional

* 1 friendly fat serving (1 to 2 tablespoons of olive oil or linseed oil to use on salads, vegetables or for cooking)

Remember: Follow one day of the Activate Cycle with a menu from the Accelerate Cycle, and alternate accordingly for a total of 17 days.

17 Sample Menus

Here are examples of how to create your daily meals during the Activate Cycle. You may follow these exactly or create your own menus based on the above guidelines. Recipes (in italics) are in the Appendix.

Wake-up drink

Every morning, as soon as you rise, drink one 240 ml (8 fl oz) cup of hot water. Squeeze half a lemon into the cup; the lemon stimulates your digestive juices. Your goal is to drink at least six to seven more glasses of water by the end of the day. The rate at which you burn calories drops if you're dehydrated. And if you're dehydrated, your body doesn't absorb nutrients properly.

Day 1

Breakfast

* 1 *Dr Mike's Power Cookie*
* 1 fresh peach, sliced
* 1 cup green tea

Lunch

* Chicken salad: baked or grilled chicken breast (diced), loose-leaf lettuce, 1 sliced tomato, assorted salad veggies, 2 tablespoons olive oil mixed with 4 tablespoons balsamic vinegar
* 115 g/4 oz brown rice
* 175 g/6 oz sugar-free fruit-flavoured yoghurt

Dinner

* Grilled salmon
* Steamed veggies

Snacks

* Protein Smoothie: 240 ml (8 fl oz) kefir blended with 115 g/4 oz frozen unsweetened berries

Day 2

* Accelerate Cycle menu

Day 3

Breakfast

* 2 scrambled egg whites
* ½ grapefruit, or other fresh fruit of your choice
* 1 cup green tea

Lunch

* 1 large bowl of *Chicken-Vegetable Soup* or grilled chicken breast and plenty of steamed veggies
* 1 medium baked potato with 1 tablespoon fat-free soured cream ('Medium' means it fits in the cup of your hand.)
* 175 g/6 oz sugar-free fruit-flavoured yoghurt
* 1 cup green tea

Dinner

* Rump steak, grilled
* Tossed salad with 1 tablespoon olive oil and 2 tablespoons balsamic vinegar
* 1 cup green tea

Snacks

* 125 g/4½ oz fresh raspberries (or other in-season fruit) with 175 g/6 oz sugar-free fruit-flavoured yoghurt
* Mediterranean spread: 125 g/4½ oz chickpeas (pureed and mixed with 1 tablespoon olive oil) and served on cucumber slices

Day 4

* Accelerate Cycle menu

Day 5

Breakfast
- 25 g/1 oz porridge oats, cooked
- 4 egg whites, scrambled
- 1 fresh peach, sliced
- 1 cup green tea

Lunch
- Prawn salad: cooked prawns, 30 g/1 oz chopped onion, generous bed of lettuce leaves, 1 tomato (large) and 1 tablespoon olive oil
- 1 baked sweet potato, medium
- 1 cup green tea

Dinner
- Pork chops, grilled
- Steamed veggies
- 1 cup green tea

Snacks
- 150 g/5 oz blueberries with 175 g/6 oz sugar-free fruit-flavoured yoghurt
- 175 g/6 oz sugar-free fruit-flavoured yoghurt or 240 ml/8 fl oz kefir

Day 6

- Accelerate Cycle menu

Day 7

Breakfast
- 2 eggs, scrambled without oil
- 1 jacket potato, diced, seasoned and browned in a small frying pan that has been coated with vegetable cooking spray
- 1 orange or other fresh fruit in season
- 1 cup green tea

Lunch
- *Turkey Black Bean Chilli*
- Large tossed salad with 1 tablespoon olive oil mixed with 2 tablespoons vinegar and seasoning
- 1 cup green tea

Dinner

* Extra lean beefburger, grilled
* Sliced fresh tomatoes, drizzled with fat-free salad dressing
* French beans or other veggie, steamed
* 1 cup green tea

Snacks

* *Kefir smoothie*
* 175 g/6 oz sugar-free fruit-flavoured yoghurt

Day 8

* Accelerate Cycle menu

Day 9

Breakfast

* 115 g/4 oz cottage cheese
* 1 medium pear, sliced
* 1 cup green tea

Lunch

* Grilled chicken breast
* 100 g/3½ oz pinto beans
* 75 g/2½ oz cooked sweetcorn
* 1 cup green tea

Dinner

* Grilled salmon
* Steamed broccoli
* Sliced fresh tomato drizzled with 1 tablespoon of olive or linseed oil mixed with vinegar and seasonings
* 1 cup green tea

Snacks

* 1 medium eating apple
* 175 g/6 oz sugar-free fruit-flavoured yoghurt

Day 10

* Accelerate Cycle menu

Day 11

Breakfast
* Kefir smoothie (blended with 115 g/4 oz berries)
* 1 cup green tea

Lunch
* Plenty of grilled beefburger
* 1 medium jacket potato
* 75 g/2½ oz peas

Dinner
* Plenty of roast turkey breast
* Steamed asparagus
* Large tossed salad with 1 tablespoon olive oil mixed with 2 tablespoons vinegar and seasoning

Snacks
* 1 medium orange
* 175 g/6 oz sugar-free fruit-flavoured yoghurt

Day 12

* Accelerate Cycle menu

Day 13

Breakfast
* 1 *Dr Mike's Power Cookie*
* 1 medium peach, sliced
* 1 cup green tea

Lunch
* *Low-Carb Primavera Delight*
* 1 cup green tea

Dinner
* Plenty of rump steak
* Large tossed salad with 1 tablespoon olive oil mixed with 2 tablespoons vinegar and seasoning
* 1 cup green tea

Snacks

- *Yoghurt Shake* (blended with fruit)
- 2nd probiotic serving of your choice

Day 14

- Accelerate Cycle menu

Day 15

Breakfast

- 85 g/3 oz Muesli or organic granola mixed with 175 g/6 oz sugar-free fruit-flavoured yoghurt (*Note:* 85 g/3 oz of Muesli gives you your 2 servings of natural starch for the day)
- 1 cup green tea

Lunch

- Fruit salad: 115 g/4 oz cottage cheese with diced fruit (85 g/3 oz diced strawberries and 85 g/3 oz diced peach) served on a generous bed of lettuce
- 1 cup green tea

Dinner

- Grilled pork chops
- Steamed or boiled cabbage
- Large tossed salad with 1 tablespoon olive oil mixed with 2 tablespoons vinegar and seasoning
- 1 cup green tea

Snacks

- 1 medium eating apple or pear
- 2nd probiotic serving of your choice

Day 16

- Accelerate Cycle menu

Day 17

Breakfast

- 2 cooked eggs (scrambled, poached, etc., without oil)
- 115 g/4 oz fresh berries
- 1 cup green tea

Lunch

- Grilled chicken breast
- 1 medium sweet potato or 150 g/5 oz mashed butternut squash
- 75 g/2½ oz cooked sweetcorn
- 1 cup green tea

(*Note:* The servings of sweet potato and/or squash plus corn
gives you your 2 servings of natural starch for the day)

Dinner

- Grilled or boiled prawns
- Steamed French beans
- Large tossed salad with 1 tablespoon olive oil mixed with 2 tablespoons vinegar and seasoning
- 1 cup green tea

Snacks

- 1 medium orange or nectarine
- 2nd probiotic serving of your choice

LEAN 17: Lost in Spice – 17 Ways to Make Veggies and Other Foods Taste Great

When you're on a diet, you've got to get creative. Here are some suggestions to get the most flavour from your food, without using added fat or sugar.

1. Basil. Basil adds loads of flavour to tomato-based dishes. It's also great with poultry.

2. Broth. Use low-sodium, low-fat chicken and beef broth to sauté meats and cook flavourful rice without adding oil.

3. Cayenne pepper. Just a pinch livens up chilli, squash and salad dressings. Consuming cayenne may help suppress your appetite. When a group of men and women took 900 milligrams of cayenne pepper half an hour before meals, they felt fuller and reduced their calorie and fat intake, according to a study appearing in the June 2005 issue of *International Journal of Obesity*.

4. Chives. Add 1 part chopped chives to 3 parts spinach and boil or steam for 3 minutes.

5. Cinnamon. Sprinkle this sweet spice in porridge, hot cereals or coffee. A 2003 study published in *Diabetes Care* reported that as little as one gram of cinnamon reduced blood glucose and cholesterol levels in type 2 diabetics.

6. Dill. Known mostly as a pickle herb, dill is delicious on fish, carrots and salads. For an easy dip, mix it into natural yoghurt and serve with cucumber slices.

7. Garlic. Stir it into mashed potatoes or salad dressing.

8. Horseradish. Ditch the gravy and go for horseradish to enliven meat. Or purée it with cottage cheese, along with some garlic and pepper, for a healthy vegetable dip or potato topping.

9. Italian seasonings (generally a combination of oregano, rosemary, savory, marjoram, basil and thyme). Sprinkle it on chicken, squash, vegetables and tomatoes.

10. Lemon. Squeeze fresh juice on salads, vegetables and fish. Grate the rind to create the zest (flavourful outer rind). This gives a tang to poultry, vegetables and salads.

11. Mint. You can't beat fresh mint from your garden, but dried mint is tasty, too. Good in tea, with fruit and in natural yoghurt.

12. Mustard. Dijon mustard adds zip to many dishes, from turkey burgers to roast potatoes.

13. Rosemary. The fragrant, needle-like leaves of this woody herb are especially good with lamb and seafood, and in any dish with beans, tomatoes, onions, potatoes or cauliflower.

14. Sage. This Mediterranean herb is especially good in tomato-based dishes, and with beans, tuna, chicken or turkey.

15. Tarragon. This wonderful seasoning makes salads and chicken taste delicious. For your salad dressings try tarragon vinegar mixed with olive oil or linseed oil.

16. Thyme. A member of the mint family, thyme is great on carrots, cauliflower, Brussels sprouts and beef.

17. Vinegar. Try cider vinegar on cooked spinach, herb or raspberry vinegar on salads, rice vinegar on chicken salad and malt vinegar on grilled fish.

SCIENCE SAYS: The Truth about High-Fructose Corn Syrup

Maybe you've heard there is controversy about high-fructose corn syrup (HFCS) in the US, which is called glucose-fructose syrup in the UK. The manufacturers say that HFCS is no worse than sugar. Well, that's like saying cigars are no worse than cigarettes. Second, they say HFCS is natural because it's made from corn. So is ethanol, and I'm not slurping down that either.

Let me set the record straight. HFCS is a cheap gooey sweetener used in soft drinks, meats, cheeses and dozens of other foods. Recent studies have raised many health concerns about the syrup. HFCS:

- Is linked to obesity. A steadily rising consumption of HFCS parallels closely with a rise in obesity. Also, HFCS very quickly turns into body fat, in some cases never even yielding energy for the body to use. One can of fizzy drink a day (the equivalent of 10 teaspoons of sugar) can lead to a 4.5 kg (10 lb) fat gain in just one year.

- Increases triglycerides, a recognised risk factor for heart disease. Also, people with elevated triglycerides overproduce a chemical component called the superoxide free radical. This molecular pickpocket can damage a variety of cell structures, including DNA, and is thought to promote ageing.

- Raises blood pressure, another risk for heart disease.

- Causes the body to over-produce insulin. High insulin is one of the earliest signs of type 2 diabetes.

- Is linked to the risk of non-alcoholic fatty liver disease. This is the most prevalent form of progressive liver disease in the US, where consumption of HFCS is exceedingly high. In this disease, the liver gets inflamed and scarred. At that point it can cause cirrhosis or liver cancer and ultimately liver failure.

- Was shown in a small study to make pancreatic cancer cells proliferate. Scientists put these cancer cells in lab dishes and fed them glucose and fructose (fructose is a sugar in HFCS). The cells gobbled up the fructose and left the glucose alone.

Should you be consuming less HFCS? Yes! Limit your intake of all added sweeteners, including HFCS, fructose, sucrose (table sugar), glucose and corn syrup. In fact, as a doctor, I'd also suggest you skip soft drinks and fruit juices altogether.

Sources: *World Journal of Gastroenterology 2010; and Cancer Research, 2010.*

Activate Cycle Worksheet

It may help you to plan your meals using the following worksheet. Using the food lists, simply fill in what you will eat each day.

Activate Day

Breakfast
Protein or probiotic serving: _____

Natural starch serving: _____

Fruit serving: _____

Lunch
Protein or probiotic serving: _____

Natural starch serving: _____

Cleansing vegetables: _____

Dinner
Protein serving: _____

Cleansing vegetables: _____

Snacks
2nd fruit serving: _____

2nd probiotic serving: _____

Other
Friendly fat serving: _____

Accelerate Days

Breakfast
Protein or probiotic serving: _____

Fruit serving: _____

Lunch
Protein or probiotic serving: _____

Cleansing vegetables: _____

Dinner

Protein serving: _____

Cleansing vegetables: _____

Snacks

2nd fruit serving: _____

2nd probiotic serving: _____

Other

Friendly fat serving: _____

Review:

- Cycle 2: Activate – is based on 'alternate day fasting', in which you alternate lower-calorie days with slightly higher-calorie days. Here you alternate Activate days with Accelerate days.

- Alternating your diet days charges up your metabolism and helps prevent dreaded weight-loss plateaus.

- Additional foods such as natural carbs are re-introduced to your diet on this Cycle.

By the time you finish the Activate Cycle, provided you've done it without cheating, you'll have enough of a weight loss that your clothes are starting to get too baggy and loose for you. Don't lose focus now, because you're doing great.

5

Cycle 3:
Achieve

· · · · · · · · · · · ·

You have been on the 17 Day Diet for 34 days now. Yes, I'm counting. We should be seeing less of you, since chips and chocolate bars are no longer padding your hips. You're looking great, fitting beautifully into clothes and, I hope, pleased with your progress.

Now is the time to start adding new food choices, including things like pasta. Pasta is not the arch-enemy of the human body, by the way. But portions the size of national monuments are. Every food group is represented on Cycle 3, and there's still an emphasis on non-starchy vegetables and lean protein. Now you can enjoy some alcohol, unless you're going to drive, you're under 18, you're pregnant, or defusing a bomb or working in a nuclear power plant.

On this Cycle, you'll eat moderately, and continue to do some form of exercise that works your cardiovascular system, only I want you to step up the duration of your workouts.

There are fewer food rules on this Cycle. However, food eaten over the sink or hob, or otherwise whilst you're standing up, still counts in your daily intake.

I call this Cycle Achieve because one of its chief purposes is to help you achieve good lifetime eating habits such as portion control, regular mealtimes and the inclusion of healthy foods.

Some of you may have already reached your goal weight, particularly if you had just 4.5 or 5.4 kg (10 or 15 lb) to take off. Congratulations. You may collect a Get-Out-of-the Achieve-Cycle-Free Card and go right to Cycle 4.

CHECK-UP: Your Progress

☐ I have lost a pleasing number of pounds.

☐ My clothes fit better.

☐ I have dropped a dress size.

☐ I have more energy.

☐ People have noticed my weight loss and complimented me.

☐ I feel more motivated to treat my body with respect.

☐ I feel less hungry.

☐ I am sleeping better.

☐ My skin looks better.

☐ My elimination has improved.

☐ My stomach is flatter.

☐ I feel lighter.

☐ I have fewer cravings.

☐ My mood is better.

For the rest of you, before we get started on Achieve Cycle 3, let's talk about what positive changes you've begun to enjoy. Look at my check-up on this page. Mark any changes that apply. Make a copy of the checklist and stick it on your fridge so that the next time you feel like nosing around in the freezer for that large pizza that you forgot to throw out, the list will stop you in your tracks.

The Speed of Weight Loss on Cycle 3

So far you have been losing weight at the speed of light, or just about. On Cycle 3 expect your weight loss to slow down a bit. I tell you this so that when you get on the scales you won't be disappointed, spoil your diet big time and vow to not start again until next January.

The goal of this Cycle is to establish healthy eating habits and produce steady, manageable weight loss. So just relax and enjoy the addition of whole-grain breads and pasta, additional fruits and vegetables, fats and snacks and alcohol in moderation (one alcoholic drink a day).

Okay, now that I've told you your weight loss may slow down a bit over the next 17 days, let me tell you how to speed it up on Cycle 3. You can do this in three ways:

1. **Increase your aerobic exercise.**

   Aerobic exercise such as walking, jogging, cycling or aerobics classes is the best way to burn fat and speed up weight loss. So if you've been doing it for at least 17 minutes a day, it's time to add even more minutes. Aim to do 45 to 60 minutes of aerobic exercise most days of the week.

2. **Continue not to eat carbs after 2.00 p.m.**

   During Cycles 1 and 2, I recommend not eating carbs after 2.00 p.m. If you did a good job of replenishing your muscle and liver glycogen throughout the day – which is what carbs do – then any excess carbs in the later afternoon and at night – a time when you're typically least active – will be readily converted to fat. On Cycle 3 you're allowed to have carbs at dinner. But if you want to spur weight loss, continue avoiding carbs after 2.00 p.m.

3. **Pass on the alcohol.**

   I know I just said you can have alcohol on Cycle 3, but please be aware that alcohol can throw a complete spanner into weight loss. Alcohol strains your liver, which responds by slowing down on functions such as fat-burning. Alcohol is also dehydrating and will cause water-weight pounds to register on the scale. If you want bigger losses on this Cycle, pass up the alcohol option.

Achieve Cycle Guidelines

1. Stay on the Achieve Cycle for 17 days.

2. Because you'll be eating more food, it's time to control your protein portions. Rather than eat protein liberally as in the two previous Cycles, keep your portions of fish, poultry and meat smaller – about the size of an average washing-up sponge. In fact, you can use that sponge to sop up any remnants of fat that might have dripped off the protein.

3. Remove skin from chicken and turkey prior to cooking or purchase skinless poultry.

DOCTOR, CAN YOU PLEASE TELL ME ?

When's the best time of day to exercise?

The short answer: the best time of day to work out is the time that works for you.

Luckily, some scientists have been working on this. However, scientists are like judges on *X Factor*. They don't agree on anything, and so their findings always conflict.

As for morning workouts, one study shows people burn 10 per cent more fat calories with early-morning workouts. Bodybuilders, who are not scientists, swear by exercising in the morning before breakfast. They claim it is the best time to shed flab. Supposedly, after a night of sleeping, your carb stores are lower, so your body is forced to go to your fat stores for fuel. But what do bodybuilders know? They only leave their exercise equipment for bodybuilding contests and more protein powder.

Most doctors will agree with me on the following: do not try pre-breakfast exercise under the following conditions: (1) if you are a diabetic or suffer from low-blood sugar, because you could become dizzy or nauseous; (2) if you are not much of a dawn's-early-light person and a morning workout sounds about as appealing as watching reruns of a reality TV programme.

As for evening workouts, a recent study by a group of Italian scientists found that women who walked in the evening burnt more fat than women who walked in the morning. It's not clear why, though.

Again, there's no bad time to exercise, except for maybe right now, when I'm hoping you're reading this chapter.

4. Trim all visible fat from meat.

5. You may eat up to two eggs a day. But don't have any more than four yolks per week if your doctor has diagnosed you with high cholesterol. Egg whites can be eaten without restriction.

6. Enjoy fresh vegetables and fruits as much as possible. For convenience frozen and canned items are fine, if chosen in moderation. Tinned and frozen fruits should be unsweetened.

7. You may have one alcoholic drink daily: 150 ml (5 fl oz) wine, 350 ml (12 fl oz) beer or 45 ml (1½ fl oz) spirits if you wish. Attention, everyone reading this: Notice I said, 'one'. If you go to a party, have one drink and spend the rest of the night drinking non-alcoholic, calorie-free drinks such as flavoured soda water. (This will help you avoid embarrassing work-party karaoke moments.) Please remember that alcohol has a dehydrating effect and can interfere with fat-burning and weight loss. One drink per day, however, has a positive effect on cholesterol levels. Accumulating evidence suggests that moderate drinking may lower the risk of heart attacks.

8. Don't eat more than two servings daily from the natural starches list.

9. Don't worry about eating all the food you're allowed each day. If you forget your second dairy or carb serving, or are too full to eat it, that's okay.

10. Eat slowly and only until full; do not overload your stomach. Use my Hunger/Fullness meter as a gauge to keep you from stuffing yourself.

11. Begin to increase your weekly aerobic exercise. Exercise for at least 150 to 300 minutes per week, depending on your physical condition (five 30-minute sessions or five 60-minute sessions).

Achieve Cycle Expanded Food List

Where indicated, add these foods to your diet, in addition to those you ate on the first 2 Cycles.

Proteins

Fish and Shellfish (from Accelerate and Activate lists)

Lean Meats (from Accelerate and Activate lists)

Poultry (from Accelerate and Activate lists, including eggs and egg whites)

Additional protein:

Quail

Pheasant

Reduced-fat turkey bacon or sausage or lunch meat

Back bacon

SCIENCE SAYS: **If You Have to Drink Alcohol on Your Diet, Drink Red Wine**

Okay, here we are back on the alcohol issue. There is some intriguing research I want to share with you about one of my favourite food groups, red wine. I mentioned earlier that red wine contains a heart-protective compound called resveratrol, which does everything but fly to the moon. Apparently, resveratrol can also reduce the number of fat cells in a person's body, and scientists think it may one day be used to treat or prevent obesity. Several years ago, researchers at the University of Ulm in Germany took a strain of human fat cell precursors, called preadipocytes. In the body these are 'baby' cells that develop into mature fat cells.

In this cell-based study they found that resveratrol inhibited the pre-fat cells from increasing and prevented them converting into mature fat cells. Also, resveratrol hindered fat storage.

This makes sense when you think about French women. French women are skinny, even though they eat a high-fat diet and drink lots of wine. In fact, according to the most recent statistics, French women also have Europe's lowest average Body Mass Index – the measure of weight that takes into account someone's height.

Scientists think the resveratrol in red wine is a fat-burner – and may be the reason why the French can eat lots of fat and still stay thin.

Source: *American Journal of Clinical Nutrition, 2010.*

Natural Starches

Breads (1 slice = 1 serving)

Cracked wheat	Pumpernickel
Fibre-enriched bread	Rye bread
Gluten-free bread	Wholegrain bagel, ½ = 1 serving
Multigrain bread	Wholegrain pitta bread, 1 pocket
Oat bran bread	Wholegrain tortilla, 25 cm (10 in)
Sugar-free bread	

High Fibre Cereals (serving)

All-Bran (55 g/2 oz)

All-Bran Extra (55 g/2 oz)

All-Bran Bran Buds (55 g/2 oz)

Fiber One (55 g/20 oz)

Gluten-free cereals
 (55 g/20 oz)

Low-sugar muesli (45 g/1½ oz)

Pasta (1 serving)

Whole-wheat pasta (55 g/2 oz)

Gluten-free pasta (55 g/2 oz)

Vegetable-based pasta (55 g/2 oz)

High-fibre pasta (55 g/2 oz)

Udon noodles (55 g/2 oz)

Vegetables and herbs – unlimited

All cleansing vegetables

Alfalfa

Broccoli sprouts

Chard

Chillies

Coriander

Courgette

Fennel

Grape leaves

Kelp and other edible seaweeds

Kohlrabi

Mange tout

Radishes

Runner beans

Rhubarb

Summer squash

Swede

Virtually any vegetable

Fruits – 2 servings daily*

Apricots

Bananas

Cherries

Currants

Figs

Kiwi

Kumquats

Guava

Mango

Papaya

Pineapple

Pomegranate

Tangerine

Virtually any fresh fruit

*Serving = 1 piece fresh or 115 g/4 oz chopped fresh fruit

Note: If you are watching your sugar intake, eat lower sugar fruits. These include apples, berries (all varieties), cherries, grapefruit, orange, peach, pear and plums.

Probiotics, Dairy and Dairy Substitutes: 1 to 2 servings daily

Note: Some people don't like dairy foods, or can't digest them properly. If you're one of them, try dairy substitutes instead (see below). Try to eat at least one serving daily from this list whilst on the Achieve Cycle.

Probiotic foods from Accelerate and Activate Cycles (1 serving)

Low-calorie cheeses: Brie, Camembert, fontina, low-fat Cheddar, Edam, feta, goat, and low-fat mozzarella (55 g/2 oz)

Low-fat cottage cheese (115 g/4 oz)

Semi-skimmed or skimmed milk (240 ml/8 fl oz)

Low-fat ricotta cheese (115 g/4 oz)

Dairy substitutes: Sugar-free rice, almond or soya milk (240 ml/8 fl oz)

Friendly Fats – 1 to 2 tablespoons daily, unless otherwise indicated

Avocado (¼ fruit = 1 serving)

Rapeseed oil (1 tablespoon = 1 serving)

Walnut oil (1 tablespoon = 1 serving)

Light mayonnaise (2 tablespoons = 1 serving)

Mayonnaise (1 tablespoon = 1 serving)

Nuts or seeds, unoiled (2 tablespoons = 1 serving)

Reduced-calorie margarines (2 tablespoons = 1 serving)

Reduced-fat salad dressings (2 tablespoons = 1 serving)

Salad dressings (1 tablespoon = 1 serving)

Trans-fat-free margarines (1 tablespoon = 1 serving)

Optional Snacks

These snacks are all under 100 calories. Plus, they're filling and fun to eat.

Babybel low-fat cheese – 2 rounds

Frozen fruit bar

Granola bar, reduced sugar and fat

Microwave popcorn, light (30 g/1 oz)

Skinny Cow ice cream

Sugar-free pudding pot

String cheese – 1 stick

Meal Planning Made Easy

Each day for the next 17 days you'll eat:

* Controlled portions of protein from an expanded list.

* Liberal amounts of vegetables from an expanded list.

* Two servings of natural starches from an expanded list.

* Two servings of fruit from an expanded list.

* One to two servings from probiotics, low-fat dairy or dairy substitutes.

* One serving of fat from an expanded list.

* Optional snacks.

* Optional daily serving of alcohol.

Here is a typical day on the Achieve Cycle:

Breakfast
* About 45 g/1½ oz hot wholegrain cereal; or 2 eggs or 4 egg whites, prepared without oil; 1 *Dr Mike's Power Cookie*; or 1 probiotic serving
* 1 fruit serving

Lunch
* Controlled portions of protein in the form of fish, shellfish, meat or chicken or eggs; or vegetables plus 1 probiotic, dairy or dairy substitute serving
* 1 serving natural starch
* Unlimited amounts of vegetables

Dinner
* Controlled portions of protein in the form of fish, shellfish, meat, or chicken or turkey
* Unlimited amounts of vegetables

SCIENCE SAYS: Liposuction Has Health Benefits

Thinking about getting liposuction? Talk to your doctor. Liposuction, like all procedures, has risks. But liposuction has been found to help reverse type 2 diabetes and reduce cholesterol.

As I mentioned earlier, obesity makes your body's cells resistant to insulin. The result is that sugar can't enter your cells, and your blood-sugar level rises. Liposuction seems to reverse that process. In a study at Brooklyn's Downstate Medical Center in New York, a surgeon removed an average of 5.4 kg (12 lb) of fat from seven young women with type 2 diabetes. After the procedure their cells lost their insulin resistance, and their blood-sugar levels dropped. The findings are intriguing. This was a small study, so it will be interesting to see if future studies into liposuction improve insulin resistance too.

The other benefit of liposuction is this: removing just 2.7 kg (6 lb) of fat can lower your cholesterol level dramatically. That's the conclusion of University of Salzburg researchers. They think sucking off just small amounts of fat shifts a patient's metabolism for the better.

Although I prefer you to help your health the old-fashioned way – diet, exercise, determination, willpower and dedication – these studies hold promise.

Snacks

* 2nd fruit serving, or
* 2nd probiotic, dairy or dairy substitute serving, or
* Food from optional snack list

Additional

* 1 serving (1 to 2 tablespoons) of friendly fat to use on salads, vegetables or for cooking)

17 Sample Menus

Here are examples of how to build menus whilst on the Achieve Cycle. You can follow these exactly or create your own.

Wake-up drink

Every morning, as soon as you rise, drink one 240 ml (8 fl oz) cup of hot water. Squeeze half a lemon into the cup; the lemon stimulates your digestive juices.

Your goal is to drink at least six to seven more glasses of water by the end of the day. The rate at which you burn calories drops if you're dehydrated. And if you're dehydrated, your body doesn't absorb nutrients properly.

Day 1

Breakfast
* 1 slice brown toast
* 1 poached, soft-boiled or hard-boiled egg
* ½ grapefruit
* 1 cup green tea

Lunch
* Chicken Caesar salad: grilled chicken breast cut in pieces, 2 handfuls of cos lettuce, other salad veggies, 2 tablespoons light Caesar dressing
* 1 slice brown toast
* 1 serving fresh fruit
* 1 cup green tea

Dinner
* Roast pork fillet
* 1–2 large handfuls of mixed salad with 2 tablespoons fat-free dressing
* 1 cup green tea

Snacks
* 1 probiotic, dairy or dairy substitute serving
* 1 frozen fruit bar

Day 2

Breakfast
* 55 g/2 oz cereal, high-fibre (i.e. All Bran or bran-based cereal)
* 240 ml/8 fl oz semi-skimmed, skimmed or soya milk or other substitute
* 115 g/4 oz fresh berries
* 1 cup green tea

Lunch
* Pitta sandwich: 1 wholegrain pitta filled with chopped lettuce and tomato; 2 tablespoons crumbled fat-free feta cheese; 1 tablespoon fat-free Italian salad dressing

- 10 baby carrots
- 1 cup green tea

Dinner
- Barbecued chicken: boneless, skinless breast with barbecue sauce, grilled or baked until done
- Steamed vegetables such as asparagus, runner beans, broccoli or cauliflower
- 1 cup green tea

Snacks
- 2nd fruit
- 1 Skinny Cow ice cream

Day 3

Breakfast
- 175 g/6 oz natural yoghurt
- 1 sliced banana
- 1 slice multigrain toast
- Sugar-free jam, 1 tablespoon (to mix with yoghurt or on toast)
- 1 cup green tea

Lunch
- Peel-and-eat prawns (boiled or steamed)
- 4 tbsp cocktail sauce
- 55 g/2 oz reduced-fat coleslaw (you can prepare a low-fat version by mixing a bag of shredded cabbage with reduced-fat mayonnaise dressing)
- 1 medium baked sweet potato
- 1 cup green tea

Dinner
- Grilled salmon
- French beans, steamed, or other veggie
- 1 cup green tea

Snacks
- 2nd fruit serving
- 2nd probiotic, dairy or dairy substitute serving

Day 4

Breakfast
* 1 *Dr Mike's Power Cookie*
* 240 ml/8 fl oz semi-skimmed, skimmed or soya milk or other substitute
* 115 g/4 oz fresh berries
* 1 cup green tea

Lunch
* Lean steak mince (browned) mixed with low-carb pasta sauce and served with 55 g/2 oz whole wheat or gluten-free pasta
* 1–2 large handfulls tossed mixed salad with 2 tablespoons reduced-fat dressing
* 1 cup green tea

Dinner
* 1 large bowl of *Chicken-Vegetable Soup*
* 1 cup green tea

Snacks
* 2nd fruit serving
* 2nd probiotic, dairy or dairy substitute serving
* 1 Skinny Cow ice cream

Day 5

Breakfast
* 2 scrambled eggs
* 2 rashers reduced-fat turkey bacon
* 115 g/4 oz fresh berries
* 1 cup green tea

Lunch
* Tuna sandwich: tuna mixed with 1 tablespoon mayonnaise, chopped celery and onion, served between two slices of whole grain bread.
* 1 fresh pear
* 1 cup green tea

Dinner
* *Low-Carb Primavera Delight*
* 1 cup green tea

Snacks
* Probiotic, dairy or dairy substitute serving
* Sugar-free pudding pot

Day 6

Breakfast
* 225 g/8 oz sugar-free fruit flavoured yoghurt
* 45 g/1½ oz Muesli or organic granola
* 1 piece fresh fruit (i.e, 1 peach, ¼ cantaloupe, ½ grapefruit or 1 orange)
* 1 cup green tea

Lunch
* Tomato stuffed with crab salad: mix lump crabmeat with 1 tablespoon light mayonnaise, 2 tablespoons chopped celery and serve on a generous bed of lettuce.
* Medium jacket potato with 1 tablespoon fat-free sour cream, or 100 g/3½ oz brown or Basmati rice
* 1 medium eating apple
* 1 cup green tea

Dinner
* Roast beef, silverside
* Courgette, sautéed with 1 tablespoon olive oil and Italian spices
* 1 cup green tea

Snack
* 2nd probiotic, dairy, or dairy substitute serving
* 1 frozen fruit bar

Day 7

Breakfast
* 115 g/4 oz low-fat or fat-free cottage cheese
* 150 g/5 oz pineapple chunks, fresh or canned in their own juice
* 1 cup green tea

Lunch
* Cheese toastie sandwich: Place 2 reduced-fat cheese slices and 2 slices tomato on 2 slices brown bread and cook in pan sprayed lightly with vegetable oil spray until toasty and cooked throughout.

* 1 cup baby carrots or other chopped fresh veggies
* 1 cup green tea

Dinner

* Baked chicken thighs, skinless
* Steamed vegetables
* 1–2 large handfuls mixed salad with 2 tablespoons reduced-fat dressing
* 1 cup green tea

Day 8

Breakfast

* 1 *Dr Mike's Power Cookie*
* 1 banana, sliced
* 1 cup skimmed milk or kefir
* 1 cup green tea

Lunch

* *Turkey Black Bean Chilli*
* 1 serving fresh fruit
* 1 cup green tea

Dinner

* Grilled salmon
* 1–2 large handfuls of mixed salad with 2 tablespoons fat-free dressing
* 1 cup green tea

Snacks

* 1 probiotic, dairy or dairy substitute serving
* 1 frozen fruit bar

Day 9

Breakfast

* 45 g/1½ oz Muesli or organic granola
* 175 g/6 oz sugar-free fruit-flavoured yoghurt
* 115 g/4 oz fresh berries
* 1 cup green tea

Lunch
* *Super Salad*
* 1 cup green tea

Dinner
* Rump steak
* 1 medium jacket potato, topped with 1 tablespoon fat-free soured cream (optional)
* Steamed vegetables such as asparagus, runner beans, broccoli or cauliflower
* 1 cup green tea

Snacks
* 2nd fruit
* 1 Skinny Cow ice cream

Day 10

Breakfast
* 25 g/1 oz porridge oats, cooked
* ½ grapefruit
* 1 cup green tea

Lunch
* *Niçoise Salad*
* 1 cup green tea

Dinner
* Baked turkey breast
* 1 medium baked sweet potato
* French beans, steamed, or other veggie
* 1 cup green tea

Snacks
* 2nd fruit serving
* 2nd probiotic, dairy or dairy substitute serving

Day 11

Breakfast
* *Spanish Omelette*
* 1 medium eating apple or pear
* 1 cup green tea

Lunch
* Lean steak mince (browned) mixed with low-carb pasta sauce and served with 55 g/2 oz whole wheat or gluten-free pasta
* 1–2 large handfuls mixed salad with 2 tablespoons reduced-fat dressing
* 1 cup green tea

Dinner
* *Sesame Fish*
* Steamed French beans
* 65 g/2½ oz acorn or butternut squash
* 1 cup green tea

Snacks
* 2nd fruit serving
* 2nd probiotic, dairy or dairy substitute serving
* 1 Skinny Cow ice cream

Day 12

Breakfast
* 4 scrambled egg whites
* 1 slice back bacon
* 175 g/6 oz melon balls
* 1 cup green tea

Lunch
* Chicken sandwich: grilled or baked chicken mixed with 1 tablespoon mayonnaise, chopped celery and onion, served between two slices of wholegrain bread.
* 1 fresh eating pear, or other fruit in season
* 1 cup green tea

Dinner

* 2 grilled lamb chops
* Steamed broccoli or cauliflower
* Cooked carrots
* 1 cup green tea

Snacks

* Probiotic, dairy or dairy substitute serving
* Sugar-free pudding pot

Day 13

Breakfast

* 240 ml/ 8 fl oz sugar-free fruit flavoured yoghurt
* 1 piece fresh fruit (i.e, 1 peach, ¼ cantaloupe, ½ grapefruit or 1 orange)
* 1 cup green tea

Lunch

* Turkey sandwich: reduced-fat turkey, 1 slice reduced-fat Emmenthal Cheese, mustard, lettuce, slice of tomato between two slices rye bread
* 1 medium eating apple
* 1 cup green tea

Dinner

* Baked chicken breast
* Courgette, sautéed with 1 tablespoon olive oil and Italian spices
* 1 cup green tea

Snack

* 2nd probiotic, dairy or dairy substitute serving
* 1 frozen fruit bar
* 1 cup green tea

Day 14

Breakfast

* 2 scrambled eggs
* 1 slice whole grain toast
* 1 cup pineapple chunks, fresh or canned in their own juice
* 1 cup green tea

Lunch
* *Lettuce Wraps*
* 1 cup green tea

Dinner
* Grilled turkey burger
* Oven-baked chips
* 1–2 large handfuls mixed salad with 2 tablespoons reduced-fat dressing
* 1 cup green tea

Day 15

Breakfast
* *Kefir Smoothie*
* 1 slice brown toast
* 1 cup green tea

Lunch
* Chicken Caesar salad: grilled chicken breast, cut in pieces; 2 handfuls cos lettuce, other salad veggies, 2 tablespoons light Caesar dressing
* 1 serving fresh fruit
* 1 cup green tea

Dinner
* Roasted pork fillet
* 1 medium sweet potato or 150 g/5 oz mashed butternut squash
* 1 cup green tea

Snacks
* 1 probiotic, dairy or dairy substitute serving
* 1 frozen fruit bar

Day 16

Breakfast
* 55 g/2 oz cereal, high-fibre (i.e. All Bran or bran-based cereal)
* 240 ml/8 fl oz semi-skimmed, skimmed or soya milk or other substitute
* 1 banana, sliced
* 1 cup green tea

Lunch
* *Taco Salad*
* 1 cup green tea

Dinner
* *Oven Barbecued Chicken*
* Steamed vegetables such as asparagus, runner beans, broccoli or cauliflower
* 1 cup green tea

Snacks
* 2nd fruit
* 1 Skinny Cow ice cream

Day 17

Breakfast
* 240 ml/8 fl oz natural yoghurt
* 115g/4 oz fresh berries
* Jam, 1 tablespoon (to mix with yoghurt)
* 1 cup green tea

Lunch
* Peel-and-eat prawns (boiled or steamed)
* 4 tbsp cocktail sauce
* 70 g/2½ oz sweetcorn
* 1 cup green tea

Dinner
* Steak
* 1 medium jacket potato with 1 tablespoon fat-free sour cream
* 1–2 handfuls mixed salad with 1 tablespoon olive oil mixed with 2 tablespoons vinegar
* 1 cup green tea

Snacks
* 2nd fruit serving
* 2nd probiotic, dairy or dairy substitute serving
* 1 fat-free pudding pot

Achieve Cycle Worksheet

It may help you to plan your meals using the following worksheet. Using the food lists simply fill in what you will eat each day.

Breakfast

Protein or probiotic or low-fat dairy serving: _____

Starch serving: _____

Fruit serving: _____

Lunch

Protein: _____

Starch serving: _____

Vegetables: _____

Dinner

Protein serving: _____

Vegetables: _____

Snacks

2nd fruit serving: _____

2nd probiotic or low-fat dairy serving: _____

Optional snack: _____

Other

Friendly fat serving: _____

If You Have More Weight to Lose

At the end of Cycle 3, if you have additional weight to lose, you have several options:

- Return to Accelerate for 17 days, continue to Activate for 17 days and follow with Achieve for 17 days, or
- Return to Activate for 17 days and follow with Achieve for 17 days, or
- Continue on with Achieve until you reach your goal weight.

Suggestion: If you are very close to your goal weight at the end of your first Achieve Cycle, it's best to return to the Accelerate Cycle for up to 17 days to reach your goal more quickly.

As we wrap up this Cycle, think for a moment about how good it feels to slim down. Replacing those lost pounds should be new-found feelings of self-control, increased health and fitness, loose clothing, continual compliments, improved physical appearance, excitement and an overall boost of pride. I know it hasn't been easy. But the accomplishment of losing weight will bring you true satisfaction – something a Happy Meal could never do.

SCIENCE SAYS: Snooze, You Lose (Weight)

Researchers are learning more about how critical sleep is to slimming down. Adequate sleep keeps important appetite and weight-loss hormones in balance so that you stay satisfied by what you eat. Lack of sleep throws off levels of these hormones. Also, people are less likely to make healthy choices when they're tired.

Doctors have a long history of missing sleep, which may explain why many doctors are fat. Being sleep-deprived goes back to our internship days when we had to stay up for 30 hours straight sometimes. Once I nodded off for a moment and almost strangled myself with my stethoscope.

If you don't have enough time to sleep at night, try to schedule at least a short power nap during the day. Napping can contribute to weight loss, according to a study in the *American Journal of Physiology, Endocrinology, and Metabolism*. (That should be great news unless you have a newborn in the house, or you're likely to be made redundant for sleeping on the job.)

Anyway, the study looked at hormone levels in 41 men and women who were part of a seven-day sleep-deprivation experiment. Those who were allowed to nap for two hours following a night without any sleep showed a significant drop in cortisol, a hormone related to high levels of stress, and weight gain around the tummy.

So forget counting calories, start counting sheep.

DOCTOR, CAN YOU PLEASE TELL ME ?

Why can't I drink diet sodas on the 17 Day Diet?

Well, you can. Just don't tell me about it.

Diet soda sure seems like a dieter's dream: you can drink as much as you want, and none of it will end up on your thighs, right? Wrong. This bubbly beverage has a sneaky mission to make you put on pounds. Here's how: diet soda is flavoured with artificial sweeteners, which can be many times sweeter than regular sugar. That super-sweet taste can instantly trigger your natural desire for high-calorie, sugary foods. The more you drink, the worse those cravings can be, prompting you to reach for real sweets. Have diet soft drinks in moderation, but concentrate more on drinking water or mineral water, which keep cravings on an even keel without sparking a junk-food binge.

Review:

* Cycle 3: Achieve is a more moderate, liberalised food plan that allows a wide range of healthy foods, eaten in proper portions for continued weight loss.

* Weight loss may slow down during Cycle 3, but you can speed it up by: (1) Increasing your aerobic exercise, (2) not eating carbohydrates of any type past 2.00 p.m., and (3) avoiding optional alcohol.

* The purpose of Cycle 3 is to help you achieve good eating habits.

6

Cycle 4:
Arrive

. . . .

You made it! Applause, everyone!

You started the 17 Day Diet, and you decided you'd do it for just 17 days. That worked wonders, so then you committed to another 17 days and another. You felt so good about yourself and proud of your achievement, that you decided to go right to your goal. By stringing those 17 day Cycles together, you reached that goal.

You fought the battle of the bulge and won! Now it's time to keep the bulge at bay, but how? With what I call the Arrive Cycle, because you've *arrived* at your goal weight. This is a huge, important accomplishment, something many people fail to do. Now, the important thing is that you stay at this weight.

At this point in the book, I have to be really, really honest and talk about a big unmentionable thing, something no one wants to acknowledge.

You will always be on some kind of diet.

You will not be able to return to your former eating habits and keep the weight off, because those very habits – like eating too many super-sized fast food meals and being inactive – created the weight in the first place. So you've always got to diet if you want to maintain this weight loss. Maintenance plans, in the dieting vernacular, really mean nothing more than following another diet.

What do you mean, I've got to diet for ever?

Yes, it's true, you've always got to watch your weight. Sorry. Keeping weight off is a bear, a big, hungry, growling one. Once a dieter, always a dieter.

Got that? Okay, so at least let's have some fun doing it.

What I propose as a 'keep-it-off strategy' is weekends off.

Let's face it: weekends have never been good for diets. You get a promotion on Friday, so you eat. Or you snuggle up to watch a video on Friday or Saturday, and you eat. Or you go out to a party, and you eat. The problem is, from 6.00 p.m. on Friday until bedtime on Sunday, your life changes. Your schedule is looser, allowing for more snacking. Then there are the social commitments. Dinners out, birthday parties, Sunday dinner – they can do you in. It seems like you need thick layers of duct tape on your mouth to prevent gorging.

Taking weekends off allows you to splurge a bit, making it easier to get back on track on Monday. Most people can be pretty disciplined Monday through Thursday, choosing meals carefully, getting in some exercise and seeing decent results on the scale. The Arrive Cycle capitalises on these normal rhythms of life and builds a *livable* maintenance plan around them.

In a nutshell here's how you keep weight off: stay strict during the week and then enjoy yourself more over the weekend. Most people do this to lose weight. I advise that you do it to keep weight off.

I'm giving you the best diet present you can have. You still eat a calorie-controlled diet during the week, then on weekends have what you like. You take off plenty of pounds, and you keep the weight off because you never get bored using my weekend principle.

The Arrive Cycle is metabolically strategic too. You can control your weight efficiently because you're shocking your metabolism back into action. Why? Because you're following five days of controlled eating, followed by two days of increased calories. By adding calories to your meals – with beefburgers, bread, ice cream, wine, cheesecake, you name it – you're speeding up your metabolism. Then, when your metabolism is roaring like a fire, you get back to your diet on Monday, burning calories faster than ever. Basically, the Arrive Cycle keeps your metabolism guessing, so it never has a chance to go into hibernation. Since your metabolism is now well trained due to better eating habits and digestive health, a few cheat treats on the weekend will not have an adverse affect.

The Arrive Cycle is not a free-for-all. You're allowed some of your favourite foods in moderation. For example: Friday night, a restaurant meal with a cocktail or two at your favourite restaurant; Saturday, pizza for lunch or dinner, plus one dessert; and Sunday, a breakfast of pancakes with maple syrup.

A good rule of thumb to follow whilst stabilising your weight is to enjoy no more than one to three 'favourite meals' each weekend.

I call this 'strategic cheating'.

I must add a warning: if the only time you aren't putting things in your mouth is whilst you're asleep, you may have an eating disorder, or a history of one. If so, this way of eating is not for you. But, 99 per cent of dieters who follow the 17 Day Diet are ready and motivated to live the Arrive Cycle, and I'll give you some super-easy strategies to make sure strategic cheating on weekends doesn't turn into pigging out during the week.

Breathe a sigh of relief. Life is about to get normal, with you locked in at a normal, healthy, beautiful weight.

Start the Arrive Cycle

The Arrive Cycle is unique in that it helps you keep your weight off, whilst letting you enjoy yourself and eat freely from your favourite foods on weekends.

Basically, the Arrive Cycle works like this:

- Monday breakfast through Friday lunch: enjoy meal plans from one of your favourite Cycles, Accelerate, Activate or Achieve.

- Friday dinner through Sunday dinner: enjoy your favourite foods and meals in moderation over the weekend.

- Enjoy no more than one to three favourite meals over the weekend. Do not binge. Eat slowly and enjoy your food.

- If desired, enjoy alcoholic drinks in moderation over the weekend (1 to 2 daily): 45 ml/1½ fl oz spirits, 150 ml/5 fl oz wine or 350 ml/ 12 fl oz beer.

- You may include soups in your daily menus, as long as they are broth-based. Avoid soups made with milk or cream. Having soup prior to a meal will help curb your appetite and help you feel full.

- As one of your fruit servings, you may substitute fruit juice (unsweetened), but no more than 175 ml/6 fl oz per serving.

- Feel free to enjoy 240 ml/8 fl oz of vegetable juice as a snack.

- Continue to use condiments in moderation. Choose low-fat, low-calorie seasonings, such as reduced-fat dressings, plus spices, herbs, lemon or lime juice, vinegar and chilli sauce.

- Exercise on weekends, as well as weekdays.

* Each Monday, I'd like you to renew your commitment to yourself and to your new incredible body. Do this, and you'll control your eating week by week, with a strategy that'll guarantee success.

The Arrive Cycle Lifestyle

Let me give you an example of how this Cycle works in real life. Mary lost 13.5 kg (30 lb) on the 17 Day Diet. To keep the weight off she follows the Accelerate Cycle Monday through Friday. For the weekends she plans meals in which she will enjoy her favourite foods. Whatever she wants the most she lets herself have on those designated weekend days. Planning is key: it is far better than spontaneous splurges.

'It was important for me to know that I had these little treats coming,' Mary says. 'But it was even more important to know that I would get right back on the 17 Day Diet on Monday, and I always did.'

Here's a look at Mary's typical week:

Monday

Breakfast
* 175 g/6 oz natural low-fat yoghurt, mixed with 115 g/4 oz berries, or other fruit (chopped)
* 1 cup green tea

Lunch
* A large salad with lots of different cleansing vegetables and some linseed dressing
* 1 medium eating apple
* 1 cup green tea

Dinner
* Plenty of grilled or baked salmon
* Liberal amounts of cleansing vegetables, steamed or raw
* 1 cup green tea

Snacks
* 175 g/6 oz sugar-free fruit-flavoured yoghurt or natural low-fat yoghurt
* Baby carrots, raw, for nibbling

Tuesday

Breakfast
* 2 scrambled eggs
* 1 medium eating pear or other fruit in season
* 1 cup green tea

Lunch
* Grilled beefburger
* Sliced or stewed tomatoes
* 1 cup green tea

Dinner
* A stir-fry of vegetables (broccoli, onions, julienne carrots, red pepper, etc.), and chicken strips with 1 tablespoon of olive oil
* 1 cup green tea

Snacks
* 115 g/4 oz fresh berries with 175 g/6 oz of yoghurt
* 1 bowl of low-fat, low-sodium chicken broth with miso (low-sodium)

Wednesday

Breakfast
* 115 g/4 oz cottage cheese
* 1 medium orange
* 1 cup green tea

Lunch
* Tuna on a generous bed of salad leaves with fat-free salad dressing
* 1 medium eating apple
* 1 cup green tea

Dinner
* Grilled chicken breast
* Steamed asparagus
* Side salad drizzled with 1 tablespoon olive or linseed oil, mixed with 2 tablespoons balsamic vinegar and seasonings
* 1 cup green tea

Snacks

* 175 g/6 oz yoghurt
* Raw, cut-up veggies, for nibbling

Thursday

Breakfast

* 2 hard-boiled or poached eggs
* ½ grapefruit or other fresh fruit in season
* 1 cup green tea

Lunch

* Baked turkey breast
* Tomatoes, sliced or stewed, drizzled with 1 tablespoon linseed oil
* 175 g/6 oz yoghurt
* 1 cup green tea

Dinner

* Grilled salmon
* Steamed French beans
* 1 cup green tea

Snacks

* 1 medium orange
* 240 ml/8 fl oz kefir or 175 g/6 oz yoghurt

Friday

Breakfast

* *Kefir Smoothie*
* 1 cup green tea

Lunch

* Grilled chicken tossed with reduced-fat salad dressing, served over a generous bed of lettuce
* 1 cup green tea

Dinner out with Friends

* Vegetable lasagne
* Tossed salad with blue cheese dressing

- Wine, two 150 ml/5 fl oz glasses
- Tiramisu, 1 serving

Snacks
- 1 medium eating apple
- 175 g/6 oz yoghurt

Saturday

Breakfast
- 2 scrambled eggs
- ½ grapefruit
- 1 cup green tea

Lunch
- Grilled salmon on a generous bed of lettuce with reduced-fat salad dressing
- 1 cup green tea

Dinner at a restaurant
- Grilled rib-eye steak
- Caesar side salad with dressing
- 1 medium baked sweet potato
- Two 150 ml/5 fl oz glasses of wine

Snacks
- 115 g/4 oz fresh berries
- 240 ml/8 fl oz kefir or 175 g/6 oz yoghurt

Sunday

Brunch
- Blueberry waffles with 2 tbsp. syrup
- 1 turkey sausage
- 1 cup of orange juice

Dinner
- Grilled chicken breast
- Steamed broccoli
- 1 cup green tea

Snacks

- 175 g/6 oz sugar-free fruit-flavoured yoghurt or plain low-fat yoghurt
- Baby carrots, raw, for nibbling

Analyse Mary's week. Note that it exemplifies a reasonable, moderate way of eating. She sticks to her diet during the week, but gives herself a little leeway on the weekends. 'Yes, I'll treat myself. I love Italian food and good wine, and I get to enjoy it on the weekends. Come Monday, I just go right back to fruits and vegetables and chicken and fish,' she says.

Mary planned her three favourite meals for the weekend. The rest of the time, she ate prudently, following the Accelerate Cycle. Mary walks briskly most days of the week and always on the weekends. There's no way she's going to regain any weight. Sometimes, she even loses weight.

The Arrive Cycle is about being healthier and smarter about your selections and not pigging out. If you want to have fried chicken on the weekends, you can. You're compensating by having healthier foods through the week. All is not lost. You don't really have to eliminate those foods. It's more about moderation and how to balance those foods in your diet with healthier meals.

Never fool yourself into thinking you can go back to your old eating habits. It is important to hang on to your new habits and eat wisely. As Mary did, all you have to do is follow your favourite Cycle, basically five days a week, then take the weekends off. And make sure you exercise.

Arrive Cycle Strategies

I want to give you a bagful of Arrive Cycle tricks to keep you going. In my experience with patients the following factors are essential for keeping the bulge at bay.

Observe the 2.25 kg (5 lb) Stop Signal

On the Arrive Cycle weigh yourself on the weekends. Anytime you see the scale register 1.4 to 2.25 kg (3 to 5 lb) over your weight goal, go right back on your favourite Cycle, Accelerate, Activate or Achieve, on Monday. Note: you'll always get back to your normal weight faster by resuming the Accelerate Cycle. If for some reason you've gained a great deal of weight (perhaps by being on holiday), your solution is to start the 17 Day Diet from the beginning and progress through all the Cycles.

I know you're saying 'ugh' right now, but hear me out. Researchers looked at thousands of people on the National Weight Control Registry in the US who had lost 27 kg (60 lb) or more and kept it off. The scientists found that 44 per cent of the subjects weighed themselves daily. You don't have to go that far, but I do recommend weekend weighing. The number you see in the morning may keep you from going overboard. One of the bedrocks of permanent weight loss is accountability, so I urge you to check the scales on both days of the weekend.

Often, busy lives take over after the 'diet', and people do not notice even large gains in weight. It's much easier to lose 1.4 kg (3 lb) than 9 kg (20 lb). Plus, studies show that people who stop weighing themselves regain weight. Don't let that happen to you!

Be a Breakfast Lover

On most diets people starve themselves in the morning so they can eat more for lunch and dinner. This doesn't work. Eat breakfast. Heck, anytime someone tells you to eat, you really should listen!

You really do need to eat breakfast. You say you're not that hungry in the morning? Okay, but eat anyway, because research shows that eating first thing will make you feel more satisfied throughout the entire day, and you'll consume fewer calories, all told. Even on weekends. What's more, I've personally found that most people who skip breakfast become ravenous by 10.30 that morning and often find themselves eating whatever is to hand, even if it's really fattening junk food.

Get on Good Terms with Salad

Have a salad when you dine out or eat at home. According to a study at Penn State University in the US, starting dinner with a large salad may help lower the number of calories you'll consume at that meal. What kind of salad are we talking about? I think you know the answer. No, not a few leaves of cos lettuce underneath a mountain of cheese and croutons. I'm talking about salad veggies topped with one tablespoon of light dressing.

Make Healthier Substitutes

Try to eat certain reduced-fat, reduced-sugar foods. These include:

- Mustard instead of mayo on sandwiches
- Skimmed or semi-skimmed milk instead of the full-fat stuff

- Low-fat spreads

- Salsa for dipping

- Reduced-sugar tomato ketchup or steak sauce

- Fat-free, sugar-free ice cream and frozen treats

- Fat-free soured cream on jacket potatoes instead of butter or soured cream

- Fat-free or reduced-calorie salad dressings

- Grilled chicken or turkey sandwiches instead of burgers at fast-food joints

Every little bit helps.

Exercise Portion Control

What's the major dietary blunder of the last ten years? Enormous portions of rice and pasta and boulder-sized potatoes and yams. Large portions and rich food in restaurants are a major source of extra calories for people following a Western-style diet, a fact not likely to change soon. (More on this in Chapter 8.) It's important to recognise this and to continue to choose well when eating out. Also, pay attention to portion sizes, and avoid help-yourself buffets where you can return for seconds ... and thirds.

Move It, Keep It Off

I said you could eat more food on the weekend, but I'm also saying you should burn off more of that food. Think about it: the weekend is when you have more time, usually, to exercise – so take advantage of your free time. Get in at least an hour of intense, heart-pumping exercise on Saturday and Sunday. If you do this, it will be a cinch to keep your weight off. Exercise is one thing that really keeps you thin and fit.

Find ways to sneak in 'lifestyle activity' too, especially on weekends. Gardening is a great example. What I see now are people sitting on riding lawnmowers with grass-catching capabilities once reserved for people with a large acreage of land to maintain. Now people are using them to mow a patch of grass the size of a bath mat. Lawn mowing is great exercise, but only if you push the mower. It burns 387 calories an hour!

Here's what other weekend chores burn per hour:

LEAN 17: 17 Weekend Chores That Incinerate Calories (per hour)

1.	Watering lawn and garden by hand	102
2.	Cleaning, dusting	176
3.	Moderate housework	246
4.	Carpentry, general	246
5.	Plumbing	246
6.	Gardening	281
7.	Bagging grass	281
8.	Raking lawn	303
9.	Weeding or planting a garden	317
10.	Painting	317
11.	Cleaning gutters	352
12.	Axe chopping, slow	362
13.	DIY	387
14.	Shovelling snow	422
15.	Moving heavy objects (like helping your child move to university)	528
16.	Farming, baling hay, cleaning barn	563
17.	Trimming trees	633

Avoid Overboard Syndrome

Never binge. Translated: no pig outs. No stuffing your face until it grows to the size of a football. Get your eating under control. Decide that this way of eating is going to change.

Make lists of trouble foods that might make you binge. Deep down, you know what these foods are, so it's best to not include them in your weekend treat meals.

Plan your week's meals in advance, so you're programming your brain and stomach to expect food. It will help you stop eating out of habit.

Stick to one of the Cycles during the week; enjoy your favourite foods on the weekends, but use your head. Go ahead and include pizza in your nutrition plan – just choose a normal portion, not a whole large pizza! Maintain that consistency, and you'll be thin for life.

No More Guilt Trips

On the Arrive Cycle, there's no need to struggle with the dieter's mentality that one bad or good deed will either break or make your weight loss efforts. You have permission to indulge – as long as it's planned and doesn't spin out of control into weekdays. You're in control; food is not in control of you. Remembering this will help you bounce back into wise eating on Monday.

And if you ever falter? Pick yourself up and get back on the programme. None of us are perfect, so there's nothing gained by putting ourselves down and returning to unhealthy, even destructive, patterns of behaviour. The healthiest option is to laugh it off and get back to business as soon as you can. Don't worry about doing it to perfection. Just do it.

Stay Focused

I often repeat the phrase 'If you always do what you always did, you'll always get what you always got.' This mantra will help you remember that if you revert to old habits, then the weight will pack right back on. Remind yourself of how great you look. Keep pictures of your new self at home, at work, even in your purse. Look at them whenever you're coming up with excuses not to exercise or considering a trip to the vending machine. Eventually you'll stop and think each time you're about to undermine your diet. In the meantime the pictures will help you to hesitate. List reasons you want to never get fat again and put them in random places next to your slim pictures. Wear tight clothing (it should fit well now) so you stop eating when you feel fat. That's a little trick one of my patients taught me.

The truth about the Arrive Cycle is that it involves more than following a diet. It's about making a permanent change in behaviour. This is a lifestyle change, a new way of living. You can now manage a lifetime of good nutrition, enjoy food and keep fat from creeping back on.

Review:

* The Arrive Cycle is the weight-stabilisation part of the 17 Day Diet.
* It provides a realistic way for you to manage your food and lifestyle.

- The foundational principle underlying the Arrive Cycle is to enjoy meal plans from one of your favourite Cycles – Accelerate, Activate or Achieve – from Monday through Friday lunch. Then Friday dinner through Sunday dinner enjoy your favourite foods and meals in moderation.

- Enjoy no more than one to three favourite meals over the weekend. Do not binge. Eat slowly and enjoy your food.

LEAN 17: 'Healthy' Foods That Will Make You Fat

Some foods with healthy reputations are actually worse for your weight than you might think. Take a look.

Food	Fattening Factor
1. Dried Fruit	Ounce for ounce, dried fruit has tons more calories than the fresh kind because it has been dehydrated and is denser. In the same volume of fresh grapes and raisins, for example, grapes have 60 calories, whilst raisins have 460.
2. Granola	It's loaded with good-for-you nuts and oats, but also with oil and sugar for more flavour. One bowl adds up to about 500 calories.
3. Muffins	Most muffins are basically just a round slice of cake. One muffin can weigh in at about 20 grams of fat, 420 calories and 34 grams of sugar.
4. Bagel	Many bagels weigh four to five ounces. At 80 calories per ounce, that's a 320- to 400-calorie hunk of bread. Stick to small, whole wheat bagels.
5. Cream	It seems harmless; after all, you pour so little over your strawberries. However, a few spoonfuls here or there over the course of a week quickly turns into 200 or more calories, plus the same amount of fat as a big knob of butter.
6. Flavoured Coffees	Drinks at the big coffee chains will sabotage your diet faster than you can say Frappuccino. Some of these items have 700 calories a serving.

table continued on the next page

Food	Fattening Factor
7. Fruit-flavoured drinks	Many bottled drinks are souped up with sugar or honey. Oh, and one bottle can contain two or more servings, bringing the calorie count to almost 200, similar to a can of soda.
8. Rice Cakes	These light snacks are fat-free and low in calories, but they're also completely lacking in fibre or protein – ingredients that can tame your hunger. That means eating two or three won't do anything, but they will add more calories to your daily total and leave you craving something with substance.
9. Fruit Juice	Juice is basically sugar and calories. A 475 ml /16 fl oz bottle of orange juice or apple juice has 55 g/2 oz of carbohydrates, the equivalent of five slices of bread. And most of that is sugar: a whopping 12 spoonfuls of it.
10. Fat-free Frozen Dessert	The label might say it's as low as 60 calories for a small pot, but lab tests on these frozen delights say otherwise: around 270 calories is more like it.
11. Reduced-fat Biscuits	Three of these will give you 150 calories. But get this: three regular chocolate-chip biscuits are 160 ... just 10 measly calories more.
12. Energy Bars	The average chocolate bar has 250 calories; so does the average energy bar. Energy bars are chocolate bars incognito, disguised by a few added vitamins (which you're better off getting from fruit). Personally, I'd rather have a Snickers.
13. Energy Drinks	The labels say they contain various herbs, minerals and the amino acid taurine, specially designed to boost your energy. But if you look at the ingredients, they're mostly caffeine and sugar, making them hardly more than overpriced squash.

Food	Fattening Factor
14. Diet Drinks	The artificial sweeteners they contain make it harder for people to regulate their calorie intake. Sweet tastes tell the brain a lot of calories are about to be consumed. When that doesn't happen, you eat more to compensate.
15. Taco Salad	One of these can weigh in at more than 900 calories (that's if you eat the hard-to-resist shell). Try my recipe for taco salad instead.
16. Trail Mix	Just 3 tablespoons of this snack packs around 140 calories. Most people gobble down much more than that, making this a very high-calorie snack.

THE 17 MINUTE WORKOUT: 17 Ways to Burn More Calories without Jogging

Activity	Effort Expended
1. Run errands	Walking briskly whilst lugging dry cleaning or groceries can burn about 120 calories in 30 minutes.
2. Fidget frequently	Research has shown that fidgeting such as tapping toes and fussing with hands blasts off up to 800 extra calories per day.
3. Get on top	Skip the passive missionary position and climb on top. This position decimates 4.5 calories per minute.
4. Take the stairs	Every minute you climb kills 7 calories.
5. Take two	Taking the stairs two at a time burns 55 per cent more calories than single stepping.
6. Rock out	Studies show that exercisers who tune in to music whilst exercising work out 25 per cent longer.
7. Give your lover a massage	An hour-long massage burns 230 calories.

table continued on the next page

Activity	Effort Expended
8. Have sex	An hour of passionate playtime kills 270 calories.
9. Pace periodically	You could burn about 100 extra calories during an 8-hour day if you walk around your office, pace whilst on your moble phone or otherwise move around.
10. Kiss	Every minute you kiss someone you burn 1 calorie.
11. Don't order take-aways	Cook at home. Spending an hour cooking burns about 150 calories. You can burn half of what you eat for dinner merely by cooking it yourself!
12. Sleep	You burn up to 200 calories whilst sleeping for around 7 hours.
13. Kick up your heels	Dancing burns 200 or more calories an hour, depending on the dance.
14. Do the hula hoop	This isn't just for kids any more. In just 10 minutes you can burn 44 calories. Plus, you tone your tummy whilst doing it.
15. Skip	Fifteen minutes of skipping burns 170 calories.
16. Play with your children	A game of hopscotch can burn 222 calories over the course of 30 minutes.
17. Coach a sports team	Coaching burns between 281 and 372 calories an hour.

THE 17 MINUTE WORKOUT: Be a Human Pretzel and Keep Weight Off

The slow stretches and meditations of yoga don't burn calories like a run on the treadmill. But a new study suggests yoga might help people *keep weight off*, especially if you're middle aged. Middle-aged people of normal weight generally put on weight over ten years, but those who did yoga gained less weight than those who didn't practise yoga.

The link between yoga and weight control has nothing to do with burning calories, since with yoga you don't actually torch much fat. Researchers believe that yoga helps keep people more in tune with their bodies and eating habits and aware of bad habits, such as eating because of stress, boredom or depression. Also, people who practise yoga tend to avoid junk food and overeating because they want to respect their bodies.

Source: *Alternative Therapies in Health and Medicine*

PART II

....

Special
Considerations

7

The 17 Day
Cultural Diet

• • • • • • • • • • • • • • • • • • •

Ilook Italian. People think I am Italian, except of course for Italians who think I'm from Brazil, Spain or Argentina. But my ancestry is Mexican; I was born and raised in the US. Because of my origins, I'm able to relate to patients from many different cultures, and because I speak Spanish I can talk to my South American patients without an interpreter in the room.

Language issues can be important in medicine. People who seek medical help but can't speak the country's predominant language sometimes find themselves getting the wrong treatment, which can turn out to be both costly and embarrassing. We had a man once who was about to be treated for back problems. But he didn't have back problems, he had constipation. He was trying to refer to his 'backside', but the nurse thought he meant 'back'. Or maybe he was too embarrassed to point to that part of his body.

In the nutrition area I feel strongly that many people, due to their heritage, are not getting adequate nutritional counselling to lose weight. This is a big problem in the US. When people come to the US from other countries, they leave their traditional foods behind and adopt the Americanised diet that is high in carbohydrates, sugar and fat – often with life-threatening consequences. Weight gain and lack of exercise, for example, are causing increased levels of heart disease and type 2 diabetes. Many people in the UK have also adopted these US dietary trends and are developing similar health problems. In both countries many of the dietary recommendations do not conform to other cultural beliefs about food or their practices. I can't solve that problem in one chapter, but I can give you a list of foods from other cultures that you can eat on all four Cycles of the 17 Day Diet. Whether you are South American, Asian, Mediterranean, Indian or Middle Eastern, or just want to experiment with other cuisines, these can be included in the 17 Day Diet.

South American Cuisine

As I know from growing up, fried food, grease and salt are common ingredients in the typical South American diet – and the cause of health-threatening disease in men, women and also children.

The good news is that if you love South American food, you don't have to turn your back on your favourites. You just need to challenge the food ingredients and preparation. Let's look at the food lists.

Cycle 1: Accelerate

Stick to the lists of approved foods, but add in these cultural selections:

Lean Proteins

Ceviche (white fish marinated in lemon juice with diced tomatoes, onions, chilli peppers and fresh coriander)

Red snapper (huachinango)

Cleansing Vegetables

Concentrate on traditional favourites such as tomatoes, onion, summer squash, cauliflower, garlic, French beans and chillies (literally hundreds of varieties), tomatillos and fresh coriander

Cycle 2: Activate

Stick to the list of approved foods, but add in these cultural selections:

Lean Proteins

Reduced-fat chorizo

Goat meat

Natural Starches

Focus on all varieties of beans and pulses

Use brown rice instead of white

Calabaza

Yucca (cassava root or manioc)

Arracache

Yautia

Plantains

Cycle 3: Achieve

Stick to the list of approved foods, but add in these cultural selections:

Lean Protein

Introduce South American-style cheese known as Queso Fresco or 'fresh cheese' as a protein. It contains less calories, fat and cholesterol than other cheeses such as Cheddar, mozzarella or processed cheese products. It's not fake cheese either, thank goodness. My idea of hell is a place where Mexican food is made with artificial cheese.

Natural Starches

Low-carb tortillas

Corn (maize) tortillas

Bollilos (sour dough bread)

Cleansing Vegetables

Chayote

Jicama

Nopales

General Tips:

* Many Mexican dishes such as beans, tortillas, Spanish rice and potatoes are good sources of carbohydrates. Beans are also high in fibre. But it is necessary to part company with tradition when it comes to frying or refrying. The time-honoured method is to fry them in fat. Try boiling instead.

* Try preparing refried beans with less oil (use olive oil, not fat), or put them through a food processor and sauté them in a pan that has been coated with vegetable oil cooking spray.

- Scale back your intake of soured cream (try Greek yogurt instead). Or use salsa or pico de gallo to top your entrees.

- Reduce fat by using a variety of cooking sprays – and for much more than just sautéing. Try butter-flavoured sprays for softening or baking tortillas, or olive oil sprays on grilled vegetables, fish or poultry.

- Use herbs and chillies in place of fats and oils.

- Use low-fat or fat-free cream cheeses. Fat-free cream cheese or low-fat ricotta lends a creamy texture to beans and sauces. Combine fat-free cream cheese and low-fat buttermilk to make a soured cream sauce. Avoid nonfat soured cream, which tends to have an offensive taste.

- Use low-fat cheeses in small amounts. They are tastier when mixed with highly flavoured ingredients like chillies, spices and salsas.

- Instead of cooking tortillas in oil or other fat, brown them on a griddle pan and then oven-bake them for a few minutes to heat the ingredients inside.

- Focus on eating simply prepared dishes flavoured with traditional seasonings minus high-carb, high-fat sauces. Salsa is another favourite made from finely diced tomatoes, onions and chilli peppers. This green or red chilli sauce adds spice to a meal but not many calories. Many South Americans are not used to eating foods without grease or salt. But with the right spices, the tastes can almost be duplicated.

Mediterranean Cuisine

There's actually no one 'Mediterranean' diet. At least 16 countries border the Mediterranean Sea. The region's cuisines include Italian, Greek and Spanish foods. Diets vary between these countries and also between regions within a country. But the common Mediterranean dietary pattern has these typical characteristics:

- High consumption of fruits and vegetables

- High consumption of bread and other cereals, potatoes, beans, nuts and seeds

- Emphasis on olive oil as an important mono-unsaturated fat source (mono-unsaturated fat doesn't raise blood-cholesterol levels the way saturated fat does)

- Low-to-moderate consumption of red meat, fish and poultry

- Low-to-moderate consumption of cheese and yoghurt

- Moderate consumption of red wine

Sounds healthy. Does a Mediterranean-style diet follow the 17 Day Diet recommendations?

Close, but not exactly. In general the diets of Mediterranean peoples contain a relatively high percentage of calories from fat. This is thought to contribute to the increasing obesity in these countries, which is becoming a concern.

For the most part the Mediterranean diet is fresh and flavoured with garlic, onions, tomatoes and fresh herbs and other vegetables. It is therefore enormously rich in antioxidants.

Most of the foods on the 17 Day Diet are found in Mediterranean cuisine. Here are few to add in.

Cycle 1: Accelerate

Stick to the lists of approved foods, but add in these cultural selections:

Cleansing Vegetables

Kale

Fennel

Flat-leaf parsley

Sugar-free pasta sauce (125 g/4½ oz = 1 serving)

Cycle 2: Activate

Adhere to the list of acceptable foods, but add in these cultural selections:

Natural Starches

Orzo

Polenta

Risotto

Tabouli (Crushed wheat kernels that have been parboiled and mixed with chopped tomatoes, parsley, mint, olive oil and lemon juice)

Cycle 3: Achieve

Stick to the list of acceptable foods, but add in these cultural selections:

Natural Starches

Flatbreads made from white wholegrain, brown and granary flour

Wholegrain Italian bread

General Tips:

- Serve hot grilled chicken on a bed of steamed broccoli rabe sprinkled with lemon juice and pepper.

- Cook liberally with canned tomatoes. Cooked tomatoes provide more beneficial antioxidants, such as cancer-fighting lycopene, than raw tomatoes.

- Stay away from fat-laden butter sauces, and stick with tomato-based veggie sauces. The calorie count will be lower.

- Try sliced fennel sautéed in a little olive oil until translucent. Add cannellini beans and top with a piece of salmon. Sprinkle with chopped flat-leaf parsley for a great Activate Cycle meal.

- Use wholegrain pasta or shirataki noodles (low-carb pasta) in place of regular pasta.

- Reduce the oil when making hummus and baba ghannoush, or delete it all together.

- Dip sliced cucumbers, rather than bread, in hummus.

- Use wholegrain pitta bread rather than white bread.

- For a nutritious, high-fibre, low-fat lunch, try wholegrain pitta bread stuffed with Greek salad.

- Heart-healthy main dishes include shish kebabs, souvlaki (Greek fast food consisting of small pieces of meat and sometimes vegetables grilled on a skewer), or plaki (fish baked or grilled with garlic and tomato sauce). Dolmas (stuffed vegetables) make an excellent choice because they are usually steamed or baked.

- For condiments: Certain spices that are popular in the Mediterranean diet – oregano, parsley and basil – can spice up your cooking, as can allium-containing vegetables such as onions and garlic.

Asian Cuisine

Asian diets are associated with the best life expectancy in the world. The longevity can be chalked up to a typical healthy, low-fat diet, which is widely believed to result in a lower frequency of heart attacks and strokes than in other countries. Asians also eat their meals at regular times, chew their food well, take in lots of fibre through vegetables and fruits and drink tea frequently. Here's how to adapt the 17 Day Diet to Asian dietary standards.

Cycle 1: Accelerate

Stick to the lists of approved foods, but add in these cultural selections:

Cleansing Vegetables

Arame, a form of kelp best known for its use in Japanese cuisine

Bamboo shoots

Beansprouts

Chinese broccoli

Dulce, sea lettuce (used in many international cuisines)

Lily pods

Mangetout

Nori, an edible seaweed commonly used as a wrap for sushi

Pak choi

Yard long beans (an Asian vegetable similar to French beans)

Cycle 2: Activate

Stick to the list of approved foods, but add in these cultural selections:

Lean Protein

Tofu, all varieties

Organic bison meat

Natural Starches

Edamame

Substitute brown rice for white rice

Cycle 3: Achieve

Natural Starches

Add in the following starches:

- Soba noodles – these distinctive Japanese noodles are made from buckwheat flour, but some whole wheat flour is usually added to strengthen the dough.
- Ramen noodles – although associated with Japan, this style of curly wheat noodles (sometimes made with egg) actually originated in China.
- Rice noodles – as the name suggests, these delicate noodles, which are used throughout South-east Asia, are made with rice flour.
- Chinese wheat noodles – a variety of noodles made from wheat and sometimes eggs.
- Udon noodles – type of wheat-flour noodle popular in Japanese cuisine.

General Tips:

- Boil, grill, steam or lightly stir-fry seafood, chicken, vegetable and tofu dishes – healthy techniques that require minimal fat.
- Try traditional steaming (often done over herb-scented water) in a multi-layered bamboo basket. You can whip up several different fat-free dishes in one pot (less hassle and washing-up) in about 10 to15 minutes. As a bonus, veggies, fish and other foods retain their shape, texture, flavours and nutrition.
- Don't deep-fry. Use a non-stick pan and spray with vegetable oil spray as needed. You'll end up getting the same effect with a fraction of the oil.
- Avoid making thick sauces laced with 'artery-popping' amounts of fat and sodium.
- Substitute tofu in recipes that call for eggs.
- Substitute turkey for beef whenever possible. Turkey has a lot less saturated fat compared to red meat. Eat more fish than meat.
- Enjoy green tea, recommended on the 17 Day Diet. It contains potent antioxidants that can lower cholesterol levels, fight heart disease, boost immune function and perhaps even destroy cancer and fat cells.
- For condiments, experiment with exotic fat-free flavours: light soy

sauce, Thai fish sauce, oyster sauce, black bean sauce, miso (fermented Japanese bean paste that is a probiotic), seaweed, chillies, wasabi (Japanese horseradish paste), kimchi (a Korean condiment made from pickled cabbage that is a probiotic), curries (favoured in Thailand), garlic, spring onions, ginger, lemongrass, basil and fresh coriander.

- What about fortune cookies? Strictly an American invention.

Indian Cuisine

Generally, Indian meals are healthy and well-balanced. They're based on a variety of antioxidant-rich vegetables; meat, fish and poultry, when included, typically come in lean cuts and small portions. Vegetarian dishes are often the centrepiece of meals too. Generally, the unique spices used in Indian dishes add flavour without fat. Here's how to adapt the 17 Day Diet to Indian dietary standards.

Cycle 1: Accelerate

Cleansing Vegetables

Sea vegetables such as arame, dulce and nori

Cycle 2: Activate

Natural Starches

Basmati rice

Red lentils

Cycle 3: Achieve

Natural Starches

Chapattis (unleavened flatbread made from brown meal)

Any type of flatbreads made from wholegrain, brown and granary flours

General Tips:

- Vegetable curries, salads with raita (shredded vegetables in natural yoghurt) and lentils make great high-fibre additions to your meals.

- Try tandoori chicken or fish for a low-fat meal with a flavorful twist.

- Use yoghurt in marinades as a tenderiser, along with ginger root, garlic and curry spices, for vegetables before grilling.

- Use yoghurt too as a low-fat substitute for cream and a thickener for curries.

- Replace ghee, a clarified butter, with olive oil or linseed oil. There is also a cholesterol-free ghee.

- Spices are an integral part of Indian cooking and alleviate the need to cook with a lot of fat. Some of the most common digestion-enhancing spices include ginger, cumin, coriander, fennel, black pepper and cinnamon. Turmeric is ubiquitous in Indian cooking and is valued for its ability to stimulate digestion, improve liver function, enhance detoxification and bolster immunity.

Middle Eastern Cuisine

Although Middle Eastern cooking may seem exotic to Westerners, its presence is felt today in our own kitchens. When we cook with oranges, pistachios, spinach or saffron, for example, we use foods that originated in the region around Persia, now called Iran. When we use basil, fresh coriander, cumin and caraway, we are drawing on an age-old tradition of meatless cooking adopted by Persians from the empires of Sumeria, Babylon, Mesopotamia and Assyria.

Middle Eastern cuisine has undergone thousands of years of refinement but has never lost touch with its roots. The home of many common herbs, the Middle East was also the source of sweet and sour sauces, stuffed vine leaves, pastries and noodles. Some historians believe that pasta originated in the Middle East, not in Italy. Worth emphasising too is that yoghurt is used widely in Middle Eastern cooking.

Here's how to adapt the 17 Day Diet to Middle Eastern dietary standards.

Cycle 1: Accelerate

Stick to the list of approved foods, but add in these cultural selections:

Cleansing vegetables

Asian aubergine

Courgette

Vine leaves

Fruits

Lemon

Sour grapes

Cycle 2: Activate

Stick to the list of approved foods, but add in these cultural selections:

Fruits

Barberries, used in Middle Eastern cooking for their sour flavour

Pomegranate

Cleansing Vegetables

Yellow peas

Probiotics

Labne, a thickened yoghurt made by straining yoghurt in muslin or a coffee filter overnight

Cycle 3: Achieve

Stick to the list of approved foods, but add in these cultural selections:

Natural Starches

Thin flat bread (lavash)

Non flatbread

General tips

- Focus on traditional dishes like torshie hazeri (blends of vinegar or lime juice and vegetables), which lend themselves well to the 17 Day Diet. Another is sabzi khordan, a plate of raw greens – green onions and watercress, mint and basil – which are eaten with the fingers, or tucked inside lavash with a slice of feta cheese.

- Sauté vegetable mixtures such as borani with a minimum of oil, or use vegetable oil cooking spray and a non-stick pan.

- Make frittatas (kuku) with egg substitutes rather than eggs to cut calories and fat.

- Use brown rice instead of white rice.

* For probiotics, enjoy classic tzatziki, a yoghurt cucumber dip made with yoghurt, grated cucumbers and garlic.

Now You're Cooking ... and Losing Weight

The 17 Day Diet works for everyone, no matter what your culture or country of origin. The main reason is that it encompasses mostly natural foods, and these are found in all cuisines. I think you have to use some food commonsense too: eating too many greasy tacos, deep-fried egg rolls or fat-laden pasta sauces can lead to increased weight, higher levels of cholesterol, clogged arteries and, ultimately, heart disease.

Fortunately, taking care of your body, health, heart doesn't have to mean giving up all your old traditional favourites. Just use low-fat cooking techniques, concentrate on fruits and vegetables in their most natural state and rely on probiotics such as yoghurt (which seems to be a staple in many cultures). Be innovative, use some ingenuity and apply some creativity, and you will lose weight.

Review

* The 17 Day Diet is adaptable to any cuisine. One reason is that it emphasises vegetables, fruits, lean protein and whole grains – food groups that are a part of all cultures.

* Food preparation is key. Using less cooking fat and fewer starchy foods, you can make-over many ethnic dishes to suit your diet.

* Be sensible: eat smaller portions and avoid frying or otherwise cooking foods in too much fat.

* The 17 Day Diet is for everyone, no matter what your cultural heritage or country of origin.

8

The PMS
Exception Diet

· ·

There's always an exception to every rule, but most of the time I want you to follow them anyway. But premenstrual syndrome (PMS) calls for bending the rules a bit.

Women, I'm sure you're happy and well-adjusted ... until a few days before your period, when you turn into Attila the Hun and snap at everyone for no apparent reason. Your family and friends avoid you, and who would blame them?

Next comes the physical stuff, like your body being so bloated that you have to go up in a clothes size. Then, as your period arrives, so do the cramps. For the next week, the love-hate relationship you have with your menstrual cycle (you love that it comes regularly; you hate everything else about it) turns hostile.

On top of all this, it's hard to stay on your diet. When you're not doubled over with cramps, you're sticking your finger in a bottle of chocolate sauce multiple times a day or eating more in one meal than Kate Moss weighs.

We doctors still aren't positive why you might get testy as your period rolls in, but the prevailing theory is that fluctuating levels of oestrogen and progesterone affect the mood-enhancing brain chemical serotonin. Serotonin is a chemical in your brain that, in proper levels, makes you feel happy. It's like a natural upper. When levels dip – which is what happens in PMS – you feel moody and grumpy.

But here's the thing: you don't have to be a slave to your menstrual cycle. You can stick to a reasonable diet that one miserable week every month – and still lose weight. This is important, because being overweight or even obese makes PMS symptoms worse. You can accomplish this by following what I call the PMS Exception Diet. It's a combination of anti-PMS foods and supplements.

There are many lucky women who don't suffer from PMS and won't need this diet. The first step, before you consider this diet, is to determine: do you suffer from PMS?

You might think that's a dumb question, and maybe it is. Most women know if they have PMS. Please humour me. We doctors went to school for eight years, and we like to put our medical training to use. We love asking questions to arrive at a diagnosis. Sometimes we even throw in a few unrelated questions, like 'What kind of shampoo do you use?' or 'Who played Carrie's California boyfriend on *Sex in the City*?'

Please take the following test. It will take just a second.

CHECK-UP: Do You Suffer from PMS?

Do you have any of these symptoms right before and/or during your period? Tick off any of the symptoms that apply.

☐ Depression	☐ Anxiety
☐ Headache	☐ Nightmares
☐ Food cravings	☐ Nausea
☐ Bloating	☐ Mood swings
☐ Cramps	☐ Breast tenderness
☐ Feelings of sadness	☐ Crying spells
☐ Desire to withdraw from social situations	☐ Sleep disturbances
☐ Irritability	☐ Hot flushes
☐ Fatigue	☐ Weight gain

It's easier to diagnose a broken arm than premenstrual syndrome, but if you have five or more of these symptoms, then you're probably suffering from PMS. Less than five, and you've probably got simple menstrual discomfort.

Whether you have emotional symptoms or yours are more physical – cravings, bloating and back pain – PMS can seem like a necessary evil. But you

DOCTOR, CAN YOU PLEASE TELL ME ❓

Aren't there any medicines my GP can prescribe for my PMS symptoms?

Women have been suffering from PMS for years, and they have been treated with tranquillisers, antidepressants and diuretics. Over-the-counter painkillers such as ibuprofen are effective against cramps. But honestly, simple changes in lifestyle (a healthy diet, exercise) have been found to be as effective as medication in eliminating symptoms.

don't have to put up with it. Armed with some cutting-edge nutritional info about this condition and a little planning, you can easily turn things around so that your period no longer has the upper hand in your life – and you can still lose weight without spoiling your diet. I'll show you how to take charge right here. First we'll look at foods that help ease symptoms, then at foods that aggravate symptoms and should be avoided and finally how to modify the 17 Day Diet for one week to help you continue losing weight.

Eat to Beat PMS

I give my female patients lists of recommendations, and I help them decide what to incorporate. Of all the changes you can make to improve your premenstrual health, doctors and nutritional experts agree that adopting healthful eating habits will have the most immediate effect. Here is an overview of what to include on the PMS Exception Diet.

Salmon and Other Fish

High in protein, fish such as salmon, tuna, halibut, sardines, mackerel and herring are also high in beneficial omega-3 fatty acids, which can decrease cramps and other symptoms. These fats also stabilise the hormone spike that makes PMS so pronounced.

One of the fatty acids in the omega-3s is DHA, short for docosahexaenoic acid. Low levels of DHA have been linked to depression. A study published in the medical journal *Lancet* stated that in regions where people ate more fish, there were fewer cases of depression. Another study, published in the *American Journal of Clinical Nutrition,* noted that the documented increase in depression in North America over the last century has paralleled the dwindling amount of DHA in our diets. Considering the evidence, I think it's a good idea to eat more fish. It seems to be a good natural treatment for depression.

Other gifts from seafood include calcium, magnesium, iron and zinc – all vital for easing symptoms.

One-Week PMS Exception Diet Prescription: aim for at least 2 to 3 servings of seafood when experiencing symptoms.

Other Lean Proteins

Enjoying lean proteins such as lean meat and chicken helps you get selenium, an important anti-PMS mineral. Anxiety is associated with a deficiency in this mineral. Five weeks after psychologists at University College in Wales started administering a daily supplement of 100 micrograms of the mineral selenium to a group of 50 women and men, the subjects reported feeling more balanced and generally in higher spirits. Those most deficient in selenium at the start reported the most dramatic mood boost. The US Department of Agriculture has reported similar findings.

Other sources of selenium are seafood (particularly tuna) and wholegrains. You can meet your entire daily selenium requirement by eating three Brazil nuts a day.

Include the following proteins this week:

Chicken breasts

Lean beef

Lean beef mince

3 Brazil nuts

One-Week PMS Exception Diet Prescription: enjoy at least 2 servings of lean protein daily. Have 3 Brazil nuts every day during your period.

Soya Proteins

Tofu, tempeh, soya milk and edamame (boiled, lightly salted soybeans in the pod) contain plant hormones called isoflavones, which may lessen PMS symptoms. There's evidence these natural compounds help your body absorb the extra oestrogen and progesterone that play a role in making you feel moody, bloated and grumpy.

One-Week PMS Exception Diet Prescription: enjoy soya foods as snacks a few times a week during your period.

Natural Carbohydrates

Carbohydrates are the dietary building blocks of serotonin, that wonderful feel-good chemical in your brain. But not all carbs seem to be equally good at building serotonin. Many women with PMS report fewer symptoms after eating complex carbohydrates (whole grains, vegetables, fruits) because they are broken down more slowly by the body, keeping blood sugar, and possibly the source of serotonin, steady. Simple carbohydrates (sugar, syrup, honey) boost your blood sugar and serotonin levels only temporarily, so after an initial high or calm, you may feel irritable or moody. Alcohol (think of it as super sugar) may have similar effects.

Carbs such as butter beans and black beans are high in potassium and magnesium – two minerals that help prevent mood swings, fatigue, cravings and bloating. Sweet potatoes are rich in the B vitamins, a family of nutrients that help curb PMS symptoms too.

One-Week PMS Exception Diet Prescription: include 3 daily servings of the following:

25 g/1 oz porridge oats, cooked

55 g/2 oz high-fibre cereal

1 slice wholegrain bread (no sugar added)

100 g/3½ oz beans or pulses

1 medium sweet potato

70 g/2½ oz sweetcorn

100 g/3½ oz barley

100 g/3½ oz brown rice

Water-flushing Vegetables

A number of foods are thought to be diuretics, meaning they help the body eliminate water. And most contain magnesium, potassium, calcium and other nutrients that can relieve PMS. Asparagus, by the way, is one of the best. It contains an amino acid called asparagine that (bonus!) acts as a diuretic to flush excess liquid out of your system. Vegetables are also full of fibre, which aids elimination and relieves abdominal bloating.

Eat the following vegetables during your period:

Asparagus

Beetroots

Cucumbers

Lettuces, all varieties

Parsley

Spinach

Tomatoes

Watercress

One-Week PMS Exception Diet Prescription: eat plenty of water-flushing vegetables liberally each day.

Higher-sugar Fruits

Like certain vegetables, many fruits are loaded with potassium, an anti-PMS nutrient. Some honourable mentions: banana, cantaloupe, grapes and mangoes. Yes, these fruits are high in sugar, but that's a plus on this plan. Fruit is nature's sweets and will help tame sugar cravings during menstruation.

Steer towards high-fibre fruits too, such as apples, pears and berries. Eat your fruit instead of drinking it, since fruit juice is almost pure sugar.

One-Week PMS Exception Diet Prescription: enjoy up to 3 servings of fresh fruits daily, with an emphasis on the fruits discussed above.

Probiotics and Calcium-rich Foods

You're already eating probiotics on the 17 Day Diet. Well, guess what? These good bacteria can keep you regular and bloat-free. In one study women with abdominal pain, bloating, constipation and/or diarrhoea who took the probiotics in supplement form for four weeks noticed less bloating than those on a placebo.

Probiotic foods such as yoghurt supply an important anti-PMS mineral: calcium. Research shows that women who consume 1000 to 1200 milligrams of calcium a day all month have fewer menstruation-related mood swings than those who skimp on dairy products. A calcium deficiency seems to make hormone fluctuations worse, so getting enough of this mineral keeps hormones steady and serotonin high. You'll feel significantly less nervous, irritable, depressed and moody.

One-Week PMS Exception Diet Prescription: enjoy 2 servings of probiotics daily. Choose from the 17 Day Diet lists.

Anti-PMS Fats

Your body needs essential fatty acids (EFAs) to efficiently metabolise hormones. EFAs are a collection of polyunsaturated fats vital for bodily functions. 'Essential' means that our body is unable to manufacture it, and we need to draw it daily from our diet.

To be of benefit to your body EFAs are converted to prostaglandins. Prostaglandins are hormone-like substances responsible for the regulation of blood pressure, dilation of blood vessels for better circulation, prevention of clotting of the blood, reduction of inflammation and regulation of insulin levels. They also act as a watchdog protecting the immune system.

Supplementation with EFAs that contain a fatty acid called gamma-linolenic acid (GLA) and/or omega-3 fats has been shown to be useful in the management of PMS symptoms. Evening primrose oil is high in GLA and is an effective anti-PMS supplement that can be taken in capsule form (see below). Linseed oil is loaded with omega-3s and is thus a great fat to eat during your period. It assists in hormonal regulation.

One-Week PMS Exception Diet Prescription: have 1 to 2 tablespoons of linseed oil daily as your friendly fat serving. Talk to your doctor about taking supplemental fats.

Chocolate

The recommendation to eat a bit of chocolate during your period is controversial. Some doctors say okay; others say no. I'm amongst those who believe that chocolate is the antidote for grumpiness. Everyone gets happy when they eat chocolate. It actually boosts the brain's production of serotonin, and chocolate contains phenylethylamine, the same brain chemical that occurs in higher concentrations when you're in love.

Chocolate has many other virtues. It's rich in magnesium, a calming mineral. If your relationship with chocolate is based on health benefits, the darker the better. Plain dark chocolate has the highest cocoa content, and cocoa is the magic stuff; it's rich in flavonoids, a group of chemicals that protect the heart and blood vessels from tissue damage. (Milk chocolate is typically sweeter and less intense than plain dark chocolate, and much lower in flavonoids.)

So go ahead, let chocolate make your day, but limit daily consumption to about 15 to 30 g (½ to 1 oz) of plain dark chocolate or some low-calorie cocoa. Of course use moderation if you feel the urge – no eating both ears off a huge chocolate bunny. Any benefit from chocolate will be spoilt if you gorge on it and gain weight. Don't deny your cravings during your menstruation, but control them.

One-Week PMS Exception Diet Prescription: enjoy 15 to 30 g (½ to 1 oz) of plain dark chocolate or some low-calorie cocoa during the week of your period if you have a craving for chocolate.

Other Nutritional Tips to Fight PMS

Multiple meals. Aim to eat five to six times (breakfast, lunch, dinner and snacks) daily. The point is to maintain a steady blood-sugar level. A steady intake of foods high in complex carbs helps keep blood sugar high, so you're less affected by the hormone-induced irritability. Try not to go more than 3 hours without eating. Meals with a good balance of natural carbohydrates and a moderate amount of protein seem to do the trick for many women.

Water your body. To avoid bloating some women steer clear of extra water right before menstruation. Putting more fluid into an already bloated body seems like the last thing you'd want to do, but in fact drinking water is one of the best ways to stimulate your body to get rid of excess fluids. (If you avoid water, your body responds by hoarding fluids, making bloating even worse.) So drink at least eight 240 ml (8 fl oz) glasses of pure water a day.

What to Avoid

A number of foods and substances will make your symptoms worse. Avoid the following.

Fizzy Drinks. You don't drink this on the 17 Day Diet, and you definitely don't want to drink them during menstruation. The bubbles in fizzy drinks will make your tummy inflate. Stick to plain water.

Gum. Chewing gum causes you to swallow excess air, and this aggravates bloating. So when someone says you're full of hot air, you are.

PM Carbs. On the 17 Day Diet you don't eat carbs past 2.00 p.m. anyway. This is a good practice to follow during menstruation. Starchy foods such as bread and pasta may cause you to retain water. Restrict them before bedtime to keep from waking up puffy.

DOCTOR, CAN YOU PLEASE TELL ME**?**

My digestion is so out of whack during my period. What can I do?

What you're describing is fairly typical. Poor digestion can actually worsen PMS, so take the following precautions:

1. Eat a variety of whole foods to ensure you get all the nutrients you need. Avoid canned, frozen and otherwise processed foods.

2. Eat freshly prepared foods whenever possible.

3. Eat your heaviest meal around noon. The later in the day you eat, the lighter your meals should be. This helps with weight control too.

4. Chewing your food thoroughly makes it easier to digest.

5. When preparing meals, create a peaceful, relaxed atmosphere in your kitchen to infuse your food with a healthful energy.

6. If possible, eat at the same time every day.

7. Eating warm or hot food promotes better digestion.

8. Don't drink cold drinks; they decrease the digestive power in your stomach. Try drinking plain hot water flavoured with freshly squeezed lemon juice.

Salt. Even a few shakes can be enough to promote bloating and breast tenderness. Cutting back on salt is a pretty easy change to make, and it can really help with your symptoms. Spice up foods with herbs, spices, low-sodium or no-salt seasonings, low-salt soy sauce, sea salt or kelp.

Caffeine. Foods and drinks containing caffeine can increase breast tenderness, anxiety, irritability and mood swings. Caffeine can also rob the body of the B vitamins, which are important for keeping hormone levels in balance. Recent studies found that the more coffee a woman drinks, the worse her PMS conditions are. Don't cut back on caffeine too drastically, or you may suffer withdrawal symptoms. Trim your coffee intake by half a cup every few days, or mix regular with decaffeinated, gradually upping the proportion of decaf over several weeks. Also begin easing up on other sources of caffeine such as some teas and colas.

Refined sugar. It's a no-no. White sugar hampers the absorption of magnesium, an important nutrient, causes large fluctuations in blood-sugar levels, which can make you feel fatigued, and robs your body of the B vitamins. Stop stuffing yourself with sugar-laced comfort foods when you're feeling low. You'll feel much better if you steer clear of sweets. The immediate lift provided by sugar is usually followed by fatigue, and if you're already susceptible to depression, then being tired may make things look worse than ever.

Alcohol. Limit your intake to no more than one drink a day, or none at all, during menstruation. It can act as a depressant and make you irritable.

Eggs. During your period, pass up eggs in favour of egg whites. The fat content in eggs can interfere with the absorption of magnesium.

The PMS Exception Diet

Here's a look at an effective way to plan your meals during your menstruation. Use these sample meals as a guideline to plan your own week of symptom-free living.

Day 1

Breakfast

- Cinnamon apple porridge: Peel and dice or grate 1 medium apple. Cook the apple with 30 g/1 oz porridge oats. Sprinkle with cinnamon and serve. Cinnamon helps stabilise blood sugar.

Lunch

- Turkey sandwich: On 2 slices wholegrain bread, spread a tablespoon of Dijon mustard and top with slices of low-fat turkey breast and tomato
- 175 g/6 oz fat-free natural or sugar-free yoghurt with 175 g/6 oz mango

Dinner

- Grilled salmon
- Large salad of lettuce, tomatoes and parsley, drizzled with 1 tablespoon of linseed oil and 2 tablespoons of herbed vinegar

Snacks

- 3 Brazil nuts
- 30 g/1 oz plain dark chocolate
- 175 g/6 oz fat-free natural or sugar-free yoghurt, or 240 ml/8 fl oz soya milk
- ½ medium cantaloupe

Day 2

Breakfast

- Cheesy parfait: Combine 115 g/4 oz cottage cheese with 115 g/4 oz berries (any variety) and 3 chopped Brazil nuts

Lunch

- 85 g/3 oz whole-wheat pasta (this constitutes your 3 servings of natural carbs for the day) topped with sugar-free pasta sauce
- 1 medium eating apple or pear

Dinner

- Grilled or baked chicken
- Plenty of steamed asparagus
- Sliced tomato, drizzled with 1 tablespoon linseed oil and herbs
- 150 g/5 oz low-fat chocolate pudding

Snacks

- 175 g/6 oz fat-free natural or sugar-free yoghurt
- 1 medium banana

Day 3

Breakfast

- 240 ml/8 fl oz cocoa made with soya milk
- 2 scrambled egg whites
- 1 slice wholegrain toast
- ½ medium cantaloupe

Lunch

- Tuna sandwich: Mix 85 g/3 oz of canned tuna with a tablespoon of light mayonnaise and 20 g/¾ oz finely diced celery. On 2 slices wholegrain bread, spread tuna mixture and top with tomato slices.
- 175 g/6 oz fat-free natural or sugar-free yoghurt with 175 g/6 oz mango

Dinner

- Grilled steak
- Large salad of lettuce, tomatoes and parsley drizzled with 1 tablespoon of linseed oil and 2 tablespoons of herbed vinegar

Snacks

- 1 medium eating apple or pear
- 3 Brazil nuts
- Large bowl of edamame

Day 4

Breakfast

- 55 g/2 oz high-fibre cereal
- 1 medium banana, sliced and served with cereal
- 240 ml/8 fl oz soya milk

Lunch

- Large spinach salad with spinach leaves, topped with 125 g/4½ oz of tofu (cubed), 2 rashers cooked turkey bacon, crumbled, 100 g/3½ oz chickpeas and chopped parsley, drizzled with fat-free dressing
- 1 slice wholegrain bread
- 175 g/6 oz fat-free natural or sugar-free yoghurt with 115 g/4 oz berries

Dinner

- Grilled pork chops
- Cucumber and tomato salad. Slice half a cucumber, combine with a few cherry tomatoes and drizzle with 1 tablespoon linseed oil and 2 tablespoons herbed vinegar.

Snacks

- 3 Brazil nuts
- 30 g/1 oz plain dark chocolate
- 175 g/6 oz fat-free natural or sugar-free yoghurt
- 1 medium eating apple or pear

Day 5

Breakfast

- Cheddar melt: Top 2 slices whole grain bread with 20 g/¾ oz grated reduced-fat Cheddar cheese. Grill until the cheese melts.
- 175 g/6 oz melon balls

Lunch

- Chef salad: Large bed of lettuce, chopped cucumber, 100 g/3½ oz chickpeas, sliced pickled beetroots and strips of baked chicken or turkey drizzled with 1 tablespoon linseed oil and 2 tablespoons herbed vinegar
- 175 g/6 oz fat-free natural or sugar-free yoghurt with 115 g/4 oz berries

Dinner

- Grilled or baked salmon
- Steamed asparagus
- 150 g/5 oz low-fat chocolate pudding

Snacks

- 175 g/6 oz fresh pineapple chunks
- 3 Brazil nuts
- Large bowl of edamame

Day 6

Breakfast

- Smoothie: in a blender, combine 120 ml/4 fl oz soya milk, 175 g/6 oz light or fat-free natural yoghurt, 1 banana, sliced, a dash of vanilla extract and 4 ice cubes
- 1 slice wholegrain toast

Lunch

- Boiled or steamed prawns
- 125 g/4½ oz butter beans
- 75 g/2½ oz sweetcorn
- 1 medium eating apple or pear

Dinner

- Grilled steak
- Mixed green salad with parsley, chopped cucumbers and cherry tomatoes, drizzled with 1 tablespoon linseed oil and 2 tablespoons seasoned or balsamic vinegar
- 150 ml/5 fl oz glass of red wine

Snacks

- 3 Brazil nuts
- 30 g/1 oz plain dark chocolate
- 175 g/6 oz fat-free natural or sugar-free yoghurt
- ½ medium cantaloupe or 175 g/6 oz strawberries

Day 7

Breakfast

- 2 scrambled egg whites
- 25 g/1 oz porridge oats, cooked
- 115 g/4 oz berries

Lunch

- Lean beefburger patty
- 200 g/7 oz brown rice
- Stewed tomatoes
- 175 g/6 oz fat-free natural or sugar-free yoghurt
- 1 medium eating apple or pear

Dinner

- Roast turkey breast
- Steamed asparagus
- Cucumber and tomato salad: slice half a cucumber, combine with a few cherry tomatoes and drizzle with 1 tablespoon linseed oil and 2 tablespoons seasoned vinegar
- 1 150 ml/5 fl oz glass of red wine

Snacks

- 3 Brazil nuts
- 30 g/1 oz plain dark chocolate
- 175 g/6 oz fat-free natural or sugar-free yoghurt
- 1 medium banana

Supplement Savvy for PMS

The tablets I do like to throw at medical problems are nutritional supplements. There are many supplements you can take on a regular basis that can help. Consult your doctor about considering the following:

Multivitamin/mineral. Take one in the morning with food. (If taking children's vitamins, take 2 tablets.) Taking a multi with food optimises the absorption of the vitamins and minerals, especially B6, magnesium and potassium – nutrients that help ease pre-menstrual distress. Vitamin B6 is important for helping the liver regulate excess oestrogen levels and has been shown to help prevent menstrual cramps.

Vitamin D. Sufficient daily intake of vitamin D (400 IU) might also alleviate PMS symptoms, particularly irritability.

Calcium carbonate. At least 1200 milligrams. The average woman's diet provides only 600 to 800 milligrams of calcium a day, not the 1000 to 1200 mg necessary to ease PMS symptoms. One study found that women who took this dose had a 48 per cent drop in the severity of their PMS symptoms. Calcium appears to enhance the brain's processing of serotonin.

Magnesium. 400 milligrams twice daily. This mineral has a calming effect and counteracts irritability. Whole grains and lentils are loaded with it, but you can also get it in a supplement. Magnesium may improve mood, and one study has shown it can provide significant relief to women suffering from menstrual headaches. Magnesium citrate, aspartate and glycinate are better absorbed than the oxide form.

Fish oil. 3 grams daily. Up your dosage to 5 grams daily when PMS symptoms begin.

Evening primrose oil. 1000 milligrams daily. It relieves one of the most common PMS symptoms: breast tenderness.

LEAN 17: 17 Bloat Busters

It's Saturday night, and you slip on your sexiest pair of jeans. One problem: your tummy is so swollen that those jeans barely zip. Sound familiar? Bloating is a common but annoying PMS symptom with many causes. Fluid retention in women is frequently due to the hormonal changes that happen right before your period arrives. There are brain hormones and brain chemicals that affect the intestinal tract; oestrogen and progesterone are actually brain chemicals. They affect the brain and nervous system, and have an effect on the motility, or movement, of the intestinal tract. Luckily, there are easy ways to banish bloat, about 17 in all. Try one of these tricks to keep your denim from fitting a little too close for comfort.

1. Stop eating high-sodium foods such as canned soups, fast food and cured meats. Sodium causes your body to hang on to water.

2. Drink more water. Believe it or not, extra fluids will help to flush out the sodium – and the bloating.

3. Avoid simple carbs (think white bread, white pasta, fries, etc.). Carbs get broken down into glucose and stored in the body as glycogen for energy. In order to be stored a water molecule must attach to that glucose. The more stored carbs you have, the heavier you'll feel.

4. Opt for high-fibre carbs such as vegetables and fruits. The longer food sits in your intestines, the more likely you are to retain water.

5. Exercise. It sweats out excess water and speeds up digestion. When you exercise, you stimulate the muscles that help move food and water through your system faster. Fight constipation by walking for at least 17 minutes each day to keep food moving through your digestive tract. Working up a sweat also releases fluids. In addition research shows that moderate exercise soothes cramps, headaches and lower-back pain, improves sleep and reduces fatigue. And exercise boosts endorphin levels, which helps improve your mood.

6. Take calcium and magnesium, as I mentioned above. Both compete with sodium for absorption into your body, so if you take in adequate amounts of either, your body is forced to flush out the salt that wasn't effectively absorbed.

7. Be wary of diuretics. When you stop taking a diuretic, your body retains more water, making you bloated for one to two weeks afterwards. This can lead to a physical dependency so that your body needs the medicine to rid itself of the excess fluid instead of doing it naturally.

8. Shun fizzy drinks. I just cannot overstate this recommendation. The caffeine in fizzy drinks dehydrates you, and phosphorus, a common additive, can inflame your intestinal wall, making you feel even puffier.

9. Discuss the appropriateness of birth control pills with your doctor. Birth control pills may stabilise your level of progesterone, a bloat-inducing hormone.

10. Boost your vitamin B6. Many PMS symptoms, including water retention, are triggered by a defect in your body's metabolism of vitamin B6. Take 50 to 100 milligrams of B6 daily to see if it helps.

11. Stop the junk. Reduce your intake of foods that are difficult to digest, such as sugary, fatty and fried fare, which can sit in your intestinal tract, causing constipation and distention.

12. Enjoy water-flushing vegetables.

13. To beat bloating try a natural diuretic drink, such as a cup of chamomile or dandelion tea or a glass of still water with lemon or lime.

14. The artificial sweetener sorbitol, found in some sugarless gums and sweets, can contribute to bloating, as can the consumption of alcohol, caffeine and even nicotine.

15. Also avoid dairy products that contain lactose – milk sugar – if they seem to worsen your bloating symptoms.

16. Up your protein intake the week before and during your menstruation. Protein has a diuretic effect on the body.

17. Take supplemental probiotics.

If the changes I'm recommending seem too daunting, try making just a few at a time. My patients tell me that eating more regularly, eliminating refined sugar and caffeine, plus exercising more, make the biggest difference. Or target your most bothersome symptoms: if your breasts really bother you, for example, try taking evening primrose oil or cutting out salt to see if you get relief.

To assess whether the PMS Exception Diet is working for you, you really have to try it for at least 6 Cycles. Keep notes. As your symptoms decrease, you'll be motivated to continue your new plan. If a symptom persists, or you keep gaining weight, consult your doctor. Keep in mind your ultimate objectives: relief of PMS symptoms and ongoing weight loss.

Review:

* Several minor adjustments in the 17 Day Diet can help you during your period. Include more omega-3 rich foods such as salmon, increase your daily intake of natural carbs to 3 servings a day, eat more water-flushing vegetables and enjoy higher-sugar fruits.

* Probiotics and calcium-rich foods help with digestion problems and mood swings.

* Eat a bit of chocolate during your period. It helps relieve stress.

* Eat often (5 to 6 daily) to maintain a steady blood-sugar level.

* Avoid fizzy drinks, chewing gum, p.m. carbs, too much salt or caffeine, refined sugar and eggs.

- Several supplements can help: a multivitamin/mineral; vitamin D, calcium, magnesium, fish oil and evening primrose oil.

- Employ bloat-busting strategies, including drinking lots of water throughout the day.

THE 17 MINUTE WORKOUT: Sunlight Soothes PMS Symptoms

Outdoor aerobic activity is best if you're trying to alleviate PMS discomfort. Sunlight has been shown to reverse depression, carbohydrate cravings, fatigue and irritability in women with PMS. Spending too much time indoors under artificial light can make PMS symptoms worse.

So try some brisk walking, playing tennis, running or cycling. These are all activities that contribute to a heightened sense of relaxation and well-being. Aerobic exercise, in general, elevates the production of endorphins – brain chemicals that have a soothing effect. It also helps keep your heart and bones healthy and relieves muscle tension.

In addition to regular aerobic activity, the next best exercise prescription for PMS includes yoga to stretch muscles, align the spine and increase mental focus. But don't overdo exercise, since excessive exercise causes irregular periods or the cessation of menstruation and unhealthful conditions that can lead to the premature loss of bone.

PART III

· · · · · · · · · · · · · · · ·

Make It Stick

9

Dining Out
on the 17 Day Diet

● ●

No one stays home any more. Where are we? We are eating out. In 2009, on average, one of every nine meals in the UK was eaten away from home. Over the past four decades, eating out has grown in popularity from 36 per cent to 60 per cent, and it now accounts for 22 per cent of our annual food and drink bill. A large portion of which could be savings if you ate at home instead. As we eat out more and more, the percentage of obese people increases, whilst their wallets decrease.

Yikes! I guess you have to ask yourself if you want to be overweight or rich.

When we dine out, most of our meals don't even include a cloth napkin because we're eating at fast food restaurants. Fast food restaurants are everywhere, even in hospitals in the US. But high-fat, high-calorie food is also served at coffee shops in UK hospitals, so you can get your health care in the same place. Hospitals claim these restaurants are not for patients, but for visitors and employees. Sure. Anyone who works in a hospital knows that a lot of that food will be smuggled into patient rooms. When you're sick in bed in the hospital, you know who your true friends are and they're not bringing flowers and balloons.

Wouldn't it be nice if hospitals got savvy and started to offer 'room service'? That's right. Meals served bedside by waiters in a black tie and crisp burgundy jackets. This would make you feel like you're in a restaurant, only you would be lying on your back in a hospital gown, staring up at the ceiling.

'Hi, my name is Walter and I'll be your waiter.'

Just when you think you get to place an order for filet mignon, garlic mash potatoes and cheesecake, Walter says:

'Would you like red, green or yellow jelly with your shepherd's pie?'

Your heart sinks and you reluctantly say, 'Red jelly'.

Regardless of where you eat out (hospitals or otherwise), you might be surprised to see just how high the calorie counts on some restaurant meals are. A fast-food burger, chips and cola can have 990 calories and some even more, and just one lonely chicken wing can be as much as 192 calories. (According to the NHS, recommended daily calorie intake for adults run from 2000 calories a day for women to 2500 calories a day for men.) So eating that burger and chips takes a huge bite out of your recommended calorie intake.

Also consider that a medium-sized Starbucks mocha coffee accompanied by a cinnamon chip scone has a whopping 770 calories, 30 grams of fat. What if you opt for a more 'healthy' carrot cake over a cheesecake? Oops. It's a whopping 560 calories for a slice (minus the coffee). These numbers aren't exactly trade secrets. You can find them on the restaurants' websites*. On the next page is a look at more calorie surprises.

Unrestrained, this type of eating out is the perfect recipe for obesity and disease down the road. But we've trained ourselves to eat out. We're just too busy too cook.

So what's the answer? Eat only steamed veggies? Refuse to dine out? On the contrary. You can dine out successfully on the 17 Day Diet and enjoy your experience by learning how to navigate any menu. These days, more restaurants than ever offer low-fat, low-cal menu items, making it easy to enjoy a delicious, nutritious dining experience if you know what to ask for. Let me offer some tips that will help you eat smart whilst dining out.

*Calorie counts at particular restaurants may vary.

Know Before You Go

With most restaurants these days, you can go online and look at their menus. See what dishes look healthy – grilled items, salads, vegetable side dishes and so forth. Decide before you go what you'll order, and stick to your decision

LEAN 17: 17 High-calorie Restaurant Choices

Menu Item	Calories*
1. Cheese chips (1 order with ranch dressing)	3010
2. Fried seafood combo platter (with 60 ml/2 fl oz tartar sauce, chips, coleslaw and 2 rolls with 2 kobs of butter)	2170
3. Fried chicken dinner, with a roll and mashed potatoes	2000
4. Combo lo mein noodle dish	1820
5. Kung Pao chicken with rice	1600
6. General Tso's chicken with rice	1600
7. Fettuccine Alfredo	1500
8. Cheesecake	1500
9. Chocolate fondant cake with ice cream	1270
10. Spaghetti with meatballs	1200
11. Beef and broccoli with rice	1200
12. Lo mein	1100
13. Stuffed potato skins (8 skins with 5 tbsp. soured cream)	1120
14. Italian super supreme pizza, indivual size	1040
15. Fast food shake, large	1010
16. Fried calamari	1000
17. Cheese quesadilla or chicken burrito	1000

once you get there. Collect the menus in the restaurants you frequent so that you have them to refer to.

Sit in a Quiet Spot

Nobody knows this, but people who sit in the more distracting parts of restaurants (by a window or in front of a TV) eat considerably more. Commotion makes it easy to lose track of how much you're putting in your mouth. If you're making a reservation, request a quiet table. If you walk in and are offered a table in a busier spot, ask for one away from the action. It's worth the wait.

Be the First to Order

You've decided to pick something light off the menu, but when your friend orders the decadent steak frites, you start to rethink your boring grilled salmon. To sidestep the temptation of your friend's less healthy dish, place your order first. If you can't order first, then make your decision, close the menu and repeat your selection to yourself to help you stick to it. If you're dining at a restaurant you visit often, just ask for your favourite healthy option without even opening the menu.

Have It Your Way

Before ordering your selections, ask the waiter about the details of the meal. This will help you make more informed choices. Some questions to ask include:

* How is this dish prepared? Can it be modified?
* What ingredients are used?
* Do you have any low-fat or low-calorie options?
* What comes with this meal?
* Can I make substitutions?
* How large are the portions?

Don't be afraid to make special requests. For example, ask for foods to be served with minimal butter, margarine or oil. Ask if a particular dish can be grilled or baked rather than fried. Also, ask that no additional salt be added to your food.

You may also be able to make substitutions. If the ingredients are on the menu, the chef should be able to accommodate your needs. A common substitution is a baked potato for chips, or a double serving of vegetables instead of a starch. If your dish does not arrive at the table the way you ordered it, don't be afraid to send it back.

If you don't see something you like, ask for it. As a paying customer you have the right to eat not only what tastes good, but what's good for you. Be 'weight assertive'!

Don't Be Seduced by Menu Descriptions

Mouth-watering descriptions such as 'tender, juicy chicken breast' or 'ripe heirloom tomatoes' are increasingly common on restaurant menus. Be aware of sensory terms such as 'velvety' mousse and nostalgic ones like 'legendary' spaghetti and meatballs. Research shows that words that promote taste and texture or appeal to diners' emotions can increase sales by 23 per cent, and can even influence the way you think the food tastes. Words like these prep your taste buds to expect your chicken to taste juicy, so to some degree it probably will.

Make a game out of picking the colourful adjectives on the menu. See who can find the most in three minutes. If you win, everyone buys you dinner. That's the rule of the game.

Stay Away from Snacking

The most damage often occurs before the actual meal begins: starter nibbles are loaded with fat. Besides that, they take away your appetite for the healthiest foods to come. Avoid them. Even the freebies such as tortilla chips and salsa at Mexican restaurants or a basket of rolls and butter at another establishment can pile up fat and calories that you don't need. If you can't exercise control, ask your waiter to remove the temptation.

Make a Meal out of Starters

Certain starters can be excellent choices for a main course. The portion size of starters is often more appropriate than the extremely large portions provided in mains. Consider healthy options such as steamed seafood, salads that aren't loaded with high-fat ingredients (such as cheese and bacon), grilled vegetables and broth-based soups. You might also choose to combine the starter with a salad; the salad will bulk up the meal so that you feel more satisfied without adding a lot of calories. Be aware that some starters, particularly fried foods or items covered in cheeses, oils and cream sauces, may be overloaded with calories and fat. Some fried starters can provide a day's worth of fat for four people!

Be Salad Savvy

A salad can be your meal's best friend or worst enemy, depending on how you toss it. Pile on fresh greens, beans and veggies, but don't drown it with high-fat dressings or toppings such as cheese, eggs, bacon or croutons. Pick calorie-friendly dressings (vinaigrettes, low-cal dressings, even a generous squeeze of fresh lemon).

Remember too that you can gain control over the fat and calories in your salad by ordering the dressing on the side. Measure out a small amount of dressing with your spoon, or with thicker salad dressing, use the fork-dipping method. Dip the tines of your salad fork in the dressing, then spear the leaves of your salad. That way, you get a taste of the dressing with each bite of salad.

If you want to be really 'good', carry a 'salad spritzer' in your handbag. Order your salad without dressing. Pull out your spritzer and spray your salad. Be aware, though, that this might scare other diners, who will think you are sanitising your salad.

And watch out for potato salads, macaroni salads, coleslaw and even tuna and chicken salads, which usually are heavy in mayonnaise, sugar and calories.

Go Low on Sides

Depending on which Cycle you're on, substitute high-calorie side dishes with low-fat options such as steamed vegetables, brown rice or fresh fruits. Forget the chips, and have baked, boiled or roast potatoes, but leave off the butter, cheese and creams. Flavour with salsa or pepper and chives instead.

Choose Low-Fat Preparation Methods

The way your main course is prepared influences its calorie and fat content. Choose grilled or baked meat. Pan-fried and deep-fried foods give you extra fat you don't need. Grilling, baking, steaming and poaching seafood, skinless poultry, lean meat and veggies give you all the flavour without all the fat.

For example, grilled chicken is lower in fat and calories than fried chicken. (If you are served chicken with skin, you can remove the skin to save significant fat and calories.)

It's not easy to get rid of all fat in restaurant meals, but have a go. Ask the waiter if the butter or oil used to prepare your dish can be reduced or eliminated. Even a grilled item may have extra fat added. For example, some grilled beef dishes call for added oil.

Enjoy Alcohol in Moderation

Drinks can be diet-killers too. Ice water is free, but fancy mixed drinks have lots of empty calories, and the alcohol can dull your reasoning. Since alcohol can contribute significant amounts of calories, limiting your intake to 150 calories worth is a good idea. The following portions of alcohol each contain 150 calories or less:

150 ml/5 fl oz wine

45 ml/1½ fl oz spirits

350 ml/12 fl oz beer

Many people find it helpful to order wine by the glass rather than the bottle so that they can better control and monitor their intake. You can decide ahead of time at which point in the meal your beverage would be most satisfying. For example, you may want to save your glass of wine for your main course and sip water whilst you wait for your meal. Holding off on alcohol until a later course also helps to decrease alcohol's effect on your inhibitions. If you drink alcohol on an empty stomach, it can relax you to the point where you lose sight of your game plan. Setting a personal limit and planning when to enjoy your drink should help you stick with your goals.

Practise Portion Control

Restaurants serve mountains of food – about two to three times the quantity that we need in a meal. This is no big secret. Just don't try to finish those mega-size portions. Consider sharing a meal or asking for left-overs to be wrapped up to take home so that you can have a quick meal at a later time. Eat until you're satisfied, not stuffed. As you're eating, use my Hunger/Fullness Meter, listen to your internal hunger signals and stop when you have had enough. Eating slowly helps you recognise such cues.

Keep track of how much you eat, and stick to the number of servings you planned to eat. You probably wouldn't take kitchen scales with you to the restaurant so that you can measure out portions, but you can rely on visual references. For example:

* A serving of cooked meat, chicken or fish is like the palm of your hand, or about the size of a deck of cards.
* A serving of green salad is like an open-cupped hand.
* A serving of fruit or vegetable is like your fist, or about the size of a tennis ball.
* A serving of jacket potato looks like a tennis ball.
* 30 g/1 oz of cheese is about the size of four stacked dice.
* A serving of salad dressing is like your thumb.
* A 85 g/3 oz beefburger is the size of a large mayonnaise jar lid.

Practise the Three-Bite Rule

Try to satisfy your sweet tooth with fresh fruits, and that's it. Wave off the dessert cart. Don't even order pudding, unless you're on Cycle 4 and are enjoying 'weekends off'.

That said, you can also practise my 'three-bite rule' with desserts if you want to watch your calories a little more strictly.

There are lots of variations on the 'three-bite rule', by the way. Mums try the three-bite rule all the time. 'Johnny, you must eat at least three bites of everything on your plate before you're excused from the table.' This usually does not work. Mothers spend many long, painful, tearful hours in a stand-off, whilst children discover at least 152 ways to say 'disgusting'.

My variation on the three-bite rule is different. If you truly want chocolate cheesecake, go ahead and have it, but limit yourself to a taste. Take three bites and then set it aside for a few minutes. You're less likely to come back to it. You might even discover that those few bites of a great dessert can be very satisfying, and might be all you really wanted in the first place. You can't possibly spoil your diet big-time on three bites of anything. After your three bites, you can ask your waiter to take it away, unless your dinner guests want to wolf it down.

Incidentally, waiters use the three-bite rule all the time. After they serve the food, they wait until you have had three bites. Then they come back and ask if everything is okay.

If you're being good on your diet, you will ask the waiter to remove the rest of the dessert. Be careful here. This may hurt his or her feelings. You have to soften the blow by explaining that you, too, are practising the three-bite rule.

Choose Wisely at Any Meal

Looking for more healthy ideas whilst dining out? These general suggestions can help you make good choices at almost any restaurant.

Breakfast

Cereal with skimmed milk topped with fruit

Porridge with fruits or raisins and skimmed milk

Brown toast

Eggs or egg whites (including omelettes)

Low-fat or 'light' yoghurt

Fresh fruits

Starters

Gazpacho or vegetable juice

Broth, bouillon or consommé

Vegetable soup without cream

Prawn cocktail

Steamed clams or mussels

Green salad (without meat or cheese) with dressing on the side

Vegetables

Steamed, stewed, boiled or grilled vegetables without butter or sauces

Starches

Jacket or boiled potatoes

Pasta or steamed rice (whole-wheat pasta and brown rice are preferable)

Main Courses

Lean meats: grilled or served au jus (trim excess fat)

Fish or skinless poultry: grilled, steamed, baked or poached in wine, lemon
juice or lime juice (all without added fat)

Drinks

Water, mineral water, soda water, tea or coffee (unsweetened)

Virgin Bloody Mary

Glass of dry red or white wine

Fast Food Choices

Grilled chicken sandwiches

Salads

Cinema Snacks

Child-sized box of popcorn

Bottle of water

Fruit (Okay, cinemas don't serve these but you can bring them in
with you. But be careful when you bite down on something juicy such as
a nectarine and spray juice on the head of the person in front of you and
create a commotion.)

Here are some other suggestions to help you choose wisely at just about any
restaurant.

Best Choices at Ethnic Restaurants

Asian	● Steamed rice
	● Steamed Chinese vegetables
	● Stir-fry vegetables with prawns/chicken
	● Teriyaki beef or chicken

	• Steamed or baked tofu (make sure it is not fried) and vegetables
	• Hot-and-sour soup
	• Miso soup
	• Dishes made with chicken or fish and vegetables
	• Steamed chicken and vegetables with a 100 g/3½ of brown rice
	• Any boiled, steamed or lightly stir-fried seafood, chicken, vegetable or tofu dishes
	• Sushi
	• Sashimi
	• Edamame
Delicatessen	• Roast turkey sandwich on multigrain bread
	• Smoked salmon with tomato and onion
	• Low-fat meats, such as low-fat turkey or even low-fat ham
	• Salad with dressing on the side
	• Brown bread, rye or pumpernickel
French	• Poached fish
	• Roasted or grilled lean meats
	• Bouillabaisse
	• Salade Niçoise
	• Broth-based soups
	• Plain vegetables
Greek/Middle Eastern	• Yoghurt-based dips
	• Meat and vegetables on a skewer
	• Grilled meat
	• Stuffed pepper with meat and rice
	• Cabbage rolls
	• Tabouleh
	• Vegetable dishes and soups

Indian	
	• Any dish with beans, rice, grains, vegetables
	• Chicken tandoori
	• Vegetable curry
	• Shrimp bhuna
	• Fish vindaloo
	• Lentil soup
	• Salad or vegetables with yoghurt dressing
Italian	
	• Minestrone
	• Vegetable antipasto
	• Mussels with pasta sauce
	• Chicken marsala
	• Clams with marinara sauce
	• Squash with pasta sauce (some Italian restaurants have sphagetti squash on their menus; it makes a delicious, low-calorie substitute for pasta)
	• Chicken cacciatore
	• Veal piccata
	• Grilled chicken or fish
Mexican	
	• Grilled foods such as chicken or fish
	• Salsa
	• Pico de gallo
	• Tortilla soup
	• Black or red beans
	• Black bean soup
	• Mexican rice
	• Chilli with beans
	• Salad, dressing on the side

Stay healthy but leave room to be flexible when you eat out: eating is an integral – and fun – part of life, and life can be unpredictable. An unexpected change in your daily eating plan isn't the end of the world. In fact, you can enjoy dining out even more if you remember that it's your total diet that counts, not individual meals. You're always going to eat out at restaurants. Hopefully, you'll eat a little differently most of the time.

Review:

- Be prepared before you go out to eat at a restaurant. Check out online menus and decide what you will order.

- Sit in a quiet spot (people eat more in noisy restaurants), and be the first to order so that you're not influenced by what your friends order.

- Be assertive with waiters. Ask how foods are prepared, and request that your order be made according to low-fat, low-calorie preparation methods.

- Make a meal out of starters, since starters portions are often smaller than main meals.

- Order salad dressing on the side, or bring your own.

- Enjoy alcohol in moderation, since it can increase your appetite and lower your inhibitions.

- Practise portion control. Don't eat the whole thing; take some home for lunch or dinner the next day.

- Try the three-bite rule, especially for puddings.

CHECK-UP: DR MIKE'S RESTAURANT QUIZ—How Much Do You Know About Nutrition at Popular Restaurants?

If you're trying to reduce the calories and fat in your diet, dining out can be a challenge. Take my quiz to test your restaurant knowledge.

1. Which 15 cm/6 in sandwich at Subway has the *fewest* calories?

   A. Subway Club

   B. Tuna

   C. Turkey Breast

   D. Spicy Italian

2. Which breakfast item at McDonald's has the *most* calories?

   A. Big Breakfast

   B. Bagel with Strawberry Jam

   C. Bacon & Egg McMuffin

   D. Bacon Roll with brown sauce

3. Which salad at Subway has the *most* calories?

   A. Black Forest Ham Salad with Fat-Free Italian Dressing

   B. Turkey Breast Salad with Fat-Free Italian Dressing

   C. Sweet Onion Chicken Teriyaki Salad with Fat-Free Italian Dressing

   D. Veggie Delite Salad with Fat-Free Italian Dressing

4. Which of these frozen desserts, of equal portions, has the *fewest* calories?

   A. no-sugar-added vanilla frozen yogurt

   B. orange sorbet

5. Of the types of pizza you can order at Pizza Hut, which variety has the *most* calories (based on 1/4 of an individual pizza)?

   A. Pepperoni Feast Pan Pizza

   B. Hawaiian Pan Pizza

   C. Chicken Supreme Pan Pizza

   D. Veggie Lover's Pan Pizza

6. What is the average calorie count of a regular vanilla shake at Burger King?

   A. 362 calories

   B. 248 calories

   C. 421 calories

   D. 195 calories

7. Which doughnut at Krispy Creme has the *most* calories?

   A. Glazed Cruller

   B. Chocolate Dreamcake

   C. Chocolate Iced Custard Filled

   D. Cinnamon Apple Filled

8. What is the *lowest*-calorie sandwich you can order at Pret A Manger?

   A. Beech Smoked BLT

   B. Lemon Chicken

   C. Cracking Egg Salad

   D. Emmenthal Salad

9. Which takeaway food has the least amount of fat?

   A. chicken korma

   B. fish and chips

   C. doner kebab

   D. pizza

10. Which grande drink (with full-fat milk) at Starbucks has the *least* calories?

   A. Cappuccino

   B. Flavoured Latte

   C. Tazo Chai Tea Latte

   D. Caffe Mocha

How did you do? The answers may surprise you:

1. The correct answer is C (Turkey Breast) at 256 calories. The Subway Club sandwich weighs in at 299 calories; the Spicy Italian sandwich, 461 calories; and the Tuna Salad sandwich, 402 calories.

2. The correct answer is A (Big Breakfast). It has 595 calories. The Bagel with Strawberry Jam has 260 calories. The Bacon Roll with brown sauce has 350 calories and the Bacon & Egg McMuffin has 340 calories.

3. The correct answer is C (Sweet Onion Chicken Teriyaki Salad with Fat-Free Italian dressing) at 235 calories. The Black Forest Ham Salad and the Turkey Breast Salad with Fat-Free Italian have 145 calories each. The Veggie Delite Salad contains 85 calories.

4. The correct answer is A (no-sugar-added vanilla frozen yogurt) at 80 calories. The orange sorbet contains 100 calories.

5. The correct answer is A (Pepperoni Feast Pan) at 227 calories. The portion of Chicken Supreme Pan Pizza has 186 calories; the Hawaiian Pan Pizza, 175; and the Vegetable Supreme Pan Pizza, 180 calories – remember these are only a quarter of the pizza made as an individual serving.

6. The correct answer is C (421 calories). The lowest calorie vanilla shake is the children's size at 290 calories; the highest calorie shake is the large chocolate shake at 635 calories.

7. The correct answer is B (Chocolate Dreamcake) at 358 calories. The Glazed Cruller has 254 calories. The Chocolate Iced Custard Filled doughnut has 307 calories and the Cinnamon Apple Filled doughnut has 269 calories.

8. The correct answer is B (Lemon Chicken). It has 370 calories. The Beech Smoked BLT has 493 calories; the Cracking Egg Salad, 439 calories; and the Emmental Salad, 494 calories.

9. The correct answer is B (fish and chips). An average portion of fish and chips has 9.42 grams per 100 g/3½ oz. The same size portion of chicken korma has 15.5 g, an average pizza 11 g and a doner kebab 16.2 g

10. The correct answer is A (Cappuccino) at 136 calories. The Flavoured Latte has 284 calories; Tazo Chai Tea Latte, 193.7 calories; and Caffe Mocha, 363.7 calories.

Source: Nutritional guides at restaurants, as of early 2011.

THE 17 MINUTE WORKOUT: Burning Off a Super Burger

Super burgers at fast food take aways can add up to almost 600 calories a serving. Here's a look at how you can burn all that off.

* Participate in a 90-minute aerobics dance class (five 17-minute cycles).
* Jog for four 17-minute cycles.
* Ride a stationary bike vigorously for four 17-minute cycles.
* Shovel snow or dig ditches for three 17-minute cycles.
* Walk moderately for eight 17-minute cycles (about 2½ hours).
* *Wouldn't it be easier NOT to eat the super burger?*

Source: Calculations are based on research data from *Medicine and Science in Sports and Exercise,* the official journal of the American College of Sports Medicine.

10

Family Challenges

Being on the 17 Day Diet can be satisfying and morale-boosting, especially as the weight melts off. But do you ever wonder how your diet might affect the people seated across the dinner table from you? You know, your loveable hubby picking at his baked chicken breast and French beans, missing the old days when lasagne wasn't banished from the kitchen?

A study published a few years ago in the *Journal of Nutrition Education and Behavior* shed some light on the plight of the dieter's significant other. Researchers interviewed 21 pairs – mostly spouses and one father-daughter duo – to understand how one person's decision to lose weight or eat healthier food affected a partner.

The good news is that for the most part, significant others saw themselves as positive influences on a partner's battle of the bulge. Other partners, however, acted more like saboteurs, refusing to alter their junk food habits, and in some cases offering little more than snide comments. A few were openly sceptical and critical of a partner's ability to succeed.

The bottom line is that your loved ones – husbands, wives, children, even your mother – may try to entice you to go off your diet even after you've made it very clear you're on it. And they may not even realise they're doing this.

There are a couple of reasons why this happens. A big one is jealousy. One person may fear that the relationship could change as a partner's waistband gets smaller, confidence grows and social life changes. It could scare your spouse that you're losing weight and developing a sexy body. He might fear that other men will find you attractive and you'll leave.

Another is fear of change. People don't want to change the status quo in their relationship. Couples often have unspoken contracts that they never articulate. For example, 'If you don't bug me about my weight, I won't bug you about your drinking. If you don't bug me about my weight, I won't bug you about smoking. If you don't bug me about my weight, I won't bug you about sex.' Then the wife decides to lose weight, and suddenly the husband says, 'Oh, my God, I'm going to have to stop smoking.'

People who sabotage do things like the following: your partner might sit down and eat a packet of biscuits right in front of you. Or refuse to touch your low-fat cuisine and demand that you make cheeseburgers. Or offer glasses of wine, and cheese and biscuits, and you fall off your weight-loss wagon night after night. Or assign himself as the watchdog of your eating habits, telling you what to eat. This controlling attitude might backfire, making you rebel and eat more (especially if he's not eating the same healthy way). It's nearly enough to end your commitment to diet and exercise, especially when someone's actions feel like personal attacks.

Of course, it's not just spouses or significant others who can throw a spanner into healthy eating regimes. Office mates or friends can be just as destructive. Often, colleagues or friends who have been unsuccessful in their own efforts to lose weight, or work mates who are competing professionally, will be unsupportive. Even so, the biggest challenges come from right under your own roof – from your family – so that's who I really want to focus on here. Finding ways to get a partner on board is important because such support can play a major role in whether you succeed or fail.

Being the only one dieting in your family is a tough situation to be in. You make up your mind – no potato crisps or chocolate ice cream in the house. No more temptations, because you're determined to change your habits and lose weight. But from talking to patients who want to lose weight, I say that's often only half the battle.

For those trying to lose weight or eat healthily, the other half – the more trying half – can be resisting your loved ones' attempts to thwart your new-found resolve. Here are some thoughts I have on the subject.

Sabotaging Remarks and How to Respond

Don't be caught off guard by someone's remarks. Here are some suggestions for responding:

Saboteur: You're wasting away. Are you sure you aren't losing too much too fast?

You: It seems that something about me being slim is concerning you (or frightening you or upsetting you). But for me, my weight loss is a good and healthy thing.

Saboteur: Are you sure you can eat that?

You: My diet is varied and healthy. I eat foods in smaller portions. Or (if such comments persist), until we can communicate about my food plan in a way that feels good to me, I don't want to discuss my diet any more.

Saboteur: You don't like my brownies all of a sudden?

You: I like your brownies very much. But I'm not hungry right now; I'm full. (Or ask to wrap up some brownies to take home, but then toss them out.)

Saboteur: Here, one doughnut left, want it?

You: I really am working hard. I'm feeling great, and it would be nice to have your support. Is there anything I can do to help you give me that?

Saboteur: It's your birthday. One piece of cake won't hurt!

You: Yes, I know. I'm just so full ... I'm going to take it home for later.

Saboteur: It's great you're losing weight. I hope you can keep it off this time.

You: You may feel that your comments about my weight are supportive, but it would help me if .... (fill in the blank with something like 'you didn't remind me of my past diets'.)

Saboteur: It's none of my business, but don't runners get a lot of knee injuries?

You: You know, I've spoken to my trainer and my exercise habits are healthy.

Saboteur: Are you still on your diet? Have you lost any weight?

You: I appreciate your questions, but I might take them as pressure and feel frustrated if I can't report better numbers every time you ask me.

Saboteur: You know, you don't seem to be the same since you lost weight.

You: I really feel confused by that comment; I really want you to be supportive of my accomplishment.

Limit Exposure to Guy Food

Are you newly married? Some newlyweds are surprised to find out that not only do their new husbands own Bart Simpson bubble bath, but also that they love junk food, and lots of it. Ice cream. Potato crisps. Foods that you may have forgotten existed, because as a single girl you often subsisted on the four basic food groups: Weight Watchers, Lean Cuisine, Healthy Choice and Slim-Fast.

Exposure to blokey junk food can tear down your defences, even if you're just trying to lose 4.5 kg (10 lb) on the 17 Day Diet. And from my experience of being a guy, I can tell you, many men do eat differently to women. The stereotypical man eats heavy, fattening food. But it is possible to lose weight whilst living with a man.

I believe you must set firm ground rules such as the fact that certain foods are out of bounds, no exceptions. Give your husband a special shelf (preferably one you can't reach) to stash his junk food. Or ask him to hide it. Out-of-sight, out-of-mind is one of the best ways of coping. Okay, every now and then, you might find some biscuits in strange places, like under the sofa cushions.

Eat Less Than He Does

Men eat more than women. It's just a fact; we eat like footballers. Even the US government has studied this: according to government surveys, the average American man 20 to 59 years old eats 2758 calories a day, whilst the average American woman 20 to 59 eats 1834 calories a day – about a third less. If you try to keep up with him, you'll keep putting on weight. Stop matching him bite for bite (you might not even know you're doing it). Always eat less than your husband does, particularly when dining out. At restaurants, immediately put one-half of your meal to one side and bring it home wrapped up.

Exercise While He Watches TV

Not only do we eat like footballers, we like to watch football on TV. Whenever you get the chance, put some exercise equipment in front of the TV and do a half hour on the stepping machine or stationary bike whilst he's watching sports. This strategy will help you get thin and stay that way.

Take Charge of the Kitchen

If your husband doesn't believe in, or think he likes, low-fat, low-cal eating, don't worry. You can make healthy foods, and he'll never know the difference (except if his trousers start getting mysteriously too baggy and loose). Instead of using all beef mince, use half turkey mince and half beef mince with spaghetti bolognese, for example. Make pasta with fresh vegetables. Cook vegetarian chilli with tons of vegetables and beans; just don't call it vegetarian. Use cooking spray to sauté foods; it's a great way to cut down on the fat and calories. Done correctly, with the right food substitutions, low-fat meals taste as good – and sometimes better – than their fattening counterparts.

Become Fitness Mates

In all seriousness the best strategy is to get healthy and fit together. As any expert will tell you, it's much easier to eat healthy, non-fattening food if everyone around you is too. You can make a big deal out of each others' success, congratulating yourselves the whole time. Enjoy mealtime conversations again instead of wolfing down food. Work out together. Invite your spouse or partner to try exercising, to try this diet or try healthy food. Phrase it lovingly: 'I want to spend more time with you because I love being together. Let's do an exercise programme together, like some couple's training or couple's yoga, or let's start cycling after work. Wouldn't that be a great opportunity to be together more often?'

The decision to get fit together marks a good time to rethink your definition of love and affection. Sometimes spouses who do most of the cooking feel that they are expressing affection by piling rich food on your plate. To resist might be translated as rejection. You've got to renegotiate here. Explain that healthy cooking accomplishes the same end: healthy cooking = love. Your 'reformed' spouse will see that coming up with non-fattening meals is a bigger present than loading you up with junk, especially when he sees all the weight you're losing and how wonderful you look. Maybe someone should think of adding a line to the wedding vows: 'For richer, for poorer ... for skinnier and chubbier ...'

By sharing the health and fitness experience with a partner, you can help each other stay motivated. Partners encourage one another to move from unhealthy to healthy behaviours. One study found that women who work out with their husbands are more likely to stick to fitness programmes than married women who exercise alone. Another found that men are three times more likely to stay on a healthy diet if their wives encourage them to do so.

Sharing the fitness experience gives you something to talk about. Better communication, especially in loving relationships, is always a source of greater closeness.

Find Other Supporters

If you've tried your best but can't get your husband or partner on board, seek help elsewhere, such as with a friend, a co-worker, other family member or hire a personal trainer. They can give you encouragement and inspiration. If you don't get any takers, join a group, such as walking club or a local yoga class. These activities are fun, and you get to meet more fitness-minded people that way.

Having positive support helps you reach your dieting and fitness goals. A team effort works more harmoniously. With two or more of you working together, there's more stamina and more motivation to get to your goals.

No matter how challenging your situation, stay focused and remember your reasons for wanting to get slimmer and healthier. Imagine if someone told you that you could live longer and have less pain in your life. Would you listen to what they had to say? Exercise and healthy eating is as close to the fountain of youth as we have today.

Review:

- Being on a diet affects the people around you. It's important for your success to bring them on board.

- Be prepared to respond to saboteurs.

- Negotiate the presence of junk food in the house with your spouse and other family members.

- Take charge of your kitchen and learn how to cook healthy meals that everyone in your family will love.

- Invite your spouse or partner to join you in your effort to get fitter.

- Build a support group of other fitness-minded people.

DOCTOR, CAN YOU PLEASE TELL ME ?

I live alone and sometimes it's hard to stay on a diet.
What suggestions do you have for me?

Single-person households have grown in recent decades to 30 per cent according to the 2001 National Census. Many single diners are deficient in calcium, iron and other important vitamins and minerals because they skip meals, snack for dinner or rely on ready meals stacked in the fridge. Eating alone can be a pleasurable and healthy activity if you plan your life around it. Some suggestions:

- Stock your kitchen with a variety of staples with a long shelf-life, such as brown rice, porridge oats and other whole grains.

- Keep to hand pre-chopped broccoli, pre-packed lettuce and yoghurt, so you don't use time as an excuse not to prepare foods.

- Make single-dish meals with all the components – grains, meat, vegetables – such as casseroles and soups. Prepare them ahead of time and freeze them so you don't have to cook a lot. Also, you can make the whole recipe but portion it into individual freezer bags.

- Take advantage of supermarket salad bars. They're a boon to single people who may have avoided fresh fruits and vegetables they couldn't use fast enough. Skip the mayonnaise-based salads and high-fat dressings, but load up on fresh vegetables and fruits. At home you can add some low-fat meat or cheese, tuna or kidney beans, and your own favourite low-fat dressing.

- Never underestimate the uses of your freezer and microwave. Bags of frozen vegetables can be a great alternative when fresh produce is not available. Rice and pasta leftovers are particularly good candidates for freezing and later use. Use your microwave for defrosting, re-heating or to speed preparation of almost any meal. Microwave dishes can often be prepared with less fat too, by adding stock or wine.

- Dinner should be pleasant, and atmosphere does contribute to a more enjoyable meal. Set the table with linens, attractive dinnerware and a centrepiece. Make a lovely meal with fresh ingredients and enjoy it with a little wine, some music on the stereo and a couple of candles. Sit at the table; don't just eat hanging over the sink.

(continued on the next page)

- If you're single, try to get together with friends on a regular schedule. Set up a Thursday night supper club and rotate homes or try a new restaurant once a month.

- Start a cooking club.

- Get together with a friend who likes to cook, and make a whole week's worth of good food and split it between you.

- Use a food delivery service and get single serving meals delivered directly to your home.

- Don't be afraid to eat out alone. I eat out most days and love experimenting. I'm quite oblivious to other diners so I don't mind being stared at. I simply open my iPad and scribble, which grabs the attention of the waiters, who think I'm a food critic.

11

Surviving Holidays

T**he holidays.** It's the time of year when the zip on your dress and the springs in your bathroom scales start getting really nervous.

That's because, for a lot of dieters, packing on weight can be a holiday tradition. Statistics on weight gain throughout the Christmas season assert that you might gain 2.25 kg (5 lb) if you don't keep your hands off the mince pies and Christmas pudding.

I started thinking about this: a 2.25 kg (5 lb) weight gain is a lot of food, if you consider that it takes 3500 calories to gain 450 g (1 lb). This means you'd have to have major binging sessions on a daily basis or eat several reindeer at a buffet. You'd also have to spend the entire holiday season on the sofa.

Still, it's easy to gain weight when you consider that the traditional Christmas dinner with starters can weigh in at more than 3000 calories!

How about this year we change that tradition? Commit to a Christmas in which you manage not to gain any weight back before it's time to resolve to lose all that weight (and so much more) yet again.

Incidentally, by 'holiday', I'm talking about everything that happens from Christmas to Easter, and everything in between including the sweetheart of all weight-gaining holidays, Valentine's Day. Holidays, however, do not include special offers at Macdonald's.

Okay, with all the office parties, cocktail receptions and dinner celebrations, can you eat, drink, be merry, stay fit and still follow the 17 Day Diet?

Answer: absolutely – by adhering to my easy-to-follow holiday strategies. If you do, there will be no need to make a get-into-shape New Year's resolution ever again. You'll start every year in super shape.

'Pre-Diet'

To prevent packing on Christmas pounds, go on the offence with 'pre-dieting'. It works like this: use the Accelerate or Activate Cycles to start trimming off a few pounds of fat before the holidays get in full swing. You can do this easily with what you've already learnt from the 17 Day Diet.

Pre-dieting has been shown in clinical trials to offset holiday weight gain. Obesity researchers in Sweden studied the effect of eating during the Christmas holidays on 46 obese patients in a weight-maintenance programme. Those dieters who had lost more than 3 kg (6½ lb) by pre-dieting during the six months prior to Christmas gained less weight (from 175 g/6 oz to 2.15 kg/ 4¾ lb) between Christmas and Epiphany (a religious festival celebrated on January 6) than those who didn't pre-diet. By contrast the patients who gained more than 3 kg (6½ lb) during the six months prior to Christmas put on an additional 2.25 kg (5 lb) on average during the holidays. The message is clear: pre-dieting clearly keeps the holiday weight from piling on.

Don't resort to any type of crash dieting, however, in which you fast or slash calories down to 700 or less a day. This can result in a loss of muscle, decreased strength and power, low energy, moodiness or irritability and compromised immunity. Stick to the Accelerate or Activate Cycles for best results.

Party Plans

The hardest part, I think, is all those parties and dinners.

At Christmas, food is everywhere. Office parties, tins packed with home-made biscuits and Christmas cake offer little escape. Not only is there more food, but it's often rich in calories, sugar and fat.

Here's what I advise for enjoying yourself, without packing on any extra weight.

- Continue the good habit of eating breakfast to help control cravings later on. (Sorry, eggnog isn't considered a good egg substitute.)

* Have healthy snacks to hand. Go for them before you treat yourself to the splurge stuff.

* Eat a healthy dinner before you go to a party. (Also, try not to eat an unhealthy dinner when you're at the party.)

* Prepare and take your own safe, low-calorie and low-fat foods to parties. That way you have at least one healthy alternative.

* Choose two or three of the healthiest starters you can find (a few prawns, some veggies or fruit, etc.) and put them on a small plate or napkin, then walk away from the table. (Keep in mind this should be two or three pieces of food, not two or three napkins or plates loaded with food.)

* Be smart at the buffet table. Fill three-quarters of your plate with vegetables and fruits, the rest with protein. (Mince pies and chocolate-covered strawberries don't count as the veggies or fruit. Stacking things as high as you can is not an acceptable method for filling your plate.) Do not circle the food table like a vulture. Serve yourself, and then go and sit down somewhere to eat.

* Avoid temptation. Just say 'no' to packaged sweets and cakes! Give them to someone who's not dieting.

* Stay away from places where snacks and goodies are offered or stored – like the canteen at work or the storecupboard at home.

* Give yourself permission to enjoy a little of everything that is usually only available during this time of year, but do it in moderation. Indulging in small amounts of Christmas treats (fruitcake being the exception) might not help you lose 9 kg (20 lb) over the holidays, but it might help you from raiding the Christmas tree for edible ornaments in the middle of the night.

* Bank your calories. Accumulate a deposit of uneaten calories on the days when you know that you will be attending parties or enjoying holiday feasts. Eat a light breakfast and lunch to save calories for later. If you're careful, the large 'withdrawal' of calories at a big dinner or event later on won't break the bank.

* Be extra good on non-party days.

* Understand the reason for the season. It's a time to celebrate good times with family and friends. Try to make the focus more on socialising and less on eating.

Fill Up on Fibre

There's an incredibly easy, no-willpower way to stay lean during the holidays, something that most of us should be doing all year but aren't: eating more fibre. Increasing your fibre intake will help to transform your Christams dieting efforts into something simple and automatic. You'll be able to keep your weight under control without working at it or driving yourself crazy.

Fibre makes you feel full, so you're less likely to stuff yourself on high-calorie foods. What's more, the fibres found in foods such as bran, wholegrain products and oats naturally bind to the fats you eat and help to escort them from the body. The net effect is a reduction in the number of calories left behind that can be stored as body fat.

So fill up on pulses, fruits and vegetables.

Manage Alcohol Consumption

At Christmas, alcohol flows like lava. Keep in mind that beer, wine and spirits are high in calories. In fact, each gram of alcohol has 7 calories, compared to 4 calories per gram for other carbs. Alcohol also stimulates your appetite. Remember too when there's alcohol in your system, the liver has to work overtime to process it, so it doesn't have adequate time to process fat. A study conducted at the University of Lausanne in Switzerland found that the

SCIENCE SAYS: Log What You Eat, Lop Off Pounds

During the holidays, keep track of what you eat and how many calories you consume daily by writing the information down in a food journal. Technically referred to as 'self-monitoring', this practice has been shown in research to promote weight loss, even during the holidays.

In one study, 38 dieters (32 women and six men) recorded their food and calorie intake during Thanksgiving, Christmas or Hanukkah and New Year's Eve. The researchers categorised the dieters into groups according to how consistently they kept track of their food and calorie consumption. Weight loss was recorded as well. The best and most consistent self-monitors lost an average of 4.5 kg (10 lb) more than the persons who had a low level of compliance with the monitoring programme.

addition of only 90 ml (3 fl oz) of alcohol per day to the diet resulted in about one third less fat being processed.

You can avoid drinking alcohol and still remain social by sipping on soda water or sparkling mineral water on the rocks with a citrus twist. Or opt for non-alcoholic beer or wine. But don't overdo it, because most of these products are high in sugar.

Fit in Exercise

This is no time to take a holiday from your workouts. Stick to your regular exercise routine. It's one of the best ways to fight fat gain during the holidays. So regardless of what comes between you and your workout, try not to eliminate it all together. If you're like most people, you'll need to let off some steam during the often-stressful holiday season, and exercise is the perfect stress reliever. Plus it helps to burn off the extra calories that you've eaten at those parties and get-togethers.

If you have the luxury of time during the holidays, why not engage in a little additional aerobics to burn off those extra calories? Do a bit more of your usual aerobic activity or try some new types just for fun. Spend an afternoon at an ice or roller-skating rink. Whack a ball around a squash court or go for a hike in the countryside.

If you're not that adventurous, try to slightly increase the duration and/or frequency of your usual aerobic exercise routine. Duration refers to the length of time that you work out. It's amazing how many additional calories you'll consume by pushing your body for just a little longer.

Another option is increasing exercise frequency: working out more times per week to incinerate more calories and fat. Add some extra weekly sessions to your normal exercise routine.

Increase your intensity. Make the effort count. For optimum fat-burning you should exercise at a level that is hard enough to raise your heart rate to 70 to 80 per cent of your maximum heart rate. (You can calculate your desired heart rate by subtracting your age from 220 and multiplying that number by 70 or 80 per cent.) As an added bonus exercising at a higher intensity has also been shown to suppress hunger.

So don't plop down on the sofa all season – move your body!

Get a Grip on Holiday Stress

I've always thought the concept of 'stress' attached to the word 'holiday' was the ultimate contradiction. Shouldn't a holiday be simply filled with joy and celebration?

Yes! Even so there is Christmas holiday stress, much of it self-imposed. What is supposed to be a time of joy and good cheer begins to resemble frantic preparations for a military invasion.

Along with the season's celebrations come temptations and preparations that can cause stress and fatigue. It's no wonder people often gain weight during this time of the year. To help you avoid the season's pitfalls, namely weight gain and stress, I'll give you my thoughts on how to organise your life to make time for what really matters. With some organisation and planning, you can sail through the season with your health and emotional well-being intact, and maybe even a few pounds lighter.

- Manage your time and priorities. To prevent being hijacked by the demands of the season, do some planning. Decide which events and activities are most important and mark your calendar accordingly, along with planning for some 'personal' time. Christmas is about family and friends, so decide which people are the most important (like family, close friends and those visiting from out of town), and spend more time with them. Gift buying and sending out Christmas cards can be overwhelming tasks. Tackling them in smaller chunks not only makes them more manageable, but more enjoyable. Try writing out several cards each evening rather than trying to do them all at once. Do your gift-buying online and avoid the annual shopping death march through toy shops, retail outlets and discount palaces.

- Guard your sleep. Stress management and overall health demand adequate sleep and should top your priority list. The best way to ensure proper rest is to set regular bedtimes. Avoid or cut down on caffeine, alcohol and tobacco; all disrupt sleeping patterns, making it difficult to drift off or stay there. Eating too much food close to bedtime adversely affects slumber as well.

- Set reasonable goals. If you want to shed fat, Christmas may not be the best time to do it. There are just too many tempting goodies around. In fact, it may be unreasonable to expect to lose any weight during the season. Maintaining your present weight, or only gaining 900 g or 1.4 kg (2 or 3 lb) instead of 3 kg (7 lb) or more, is a more sensible goal.

* Cancel the guilt trips. If, after all your planning and commitment, you do overindulge, try not to feel guilty. Guilt only weakens your resolve to maintain healthy habits. Besides, guilt can spoil the fun of your celebrations, and this is a time of year to be merry. Even if you do veer off your programme, don't let that be your downfall. See the bigger picture without worrying about every little deviation from your plan. Simply do the next healthy thing for yourself: exercise, have a nutritious meal or do some relaxation exercises.

* Be of good cheer. Send a contribution to someone in need, volunteer at a shelter or contribute to a charity. Take a few moments of each day to simply say thank you for what you have. Release anger, bitterness and resentment. Be like a child again in how you view the season; it will help you live with more wonder and enthusiasm. And finally, hold each day sacred. The present is the greatest gift of all.

If you take just a few pieces of my advice, I doubt if you'll have even one vision of a sugar plum or be tempted to sneak a mince pie.

Review:

* Pre-diet before Christmas. That way, you'll start off weighing less. Should you gain weight over the holidays, it won't be such as big deal.
* Eat strategically at parties and holiday gatherings so you don't go overboard.
* Fill up on fibre-rich foods to keep from overeating.
* Keep track of what you eat by writing it down.
* Don't neglect exercise.
* Use stress-reducing techniques.
* Remember the real reason behind the season.

LEAN 17: The 17 Most Fattening Holiday Foods and How to Downsize Them

H ere are 17 holiday favourites from around the world. Note how they stack up calorie-wise and what you can do to soften the blow.

Food	Calories per Serving	The Leaner Eat
1. 225 g/8-oz cheese ball	729	Opt for reduced-calorie cheese as a starter.
2. Eggnog (265 ml/9 fl oz)	343	Make your own low-fat version with egg substitute, lite evaporated milk, rum extract and some natural low-calorie sweetener.
3. Dinner rolls	84 to 201	Serve brown rolls or no bread at all.
4. Cranberry sauce (125 g/4½ oz)	223	Serve reduced-sugar cranberry sauce and save around 150 calories.
5. Candied yams (135 g/4¾ oz)	420	Mash sweet potatoes with a little orange juice; omit the sugar and marshmallows.
6. Mashed potatoes and gravy, large helping	240	Mash 2 parts potatoes and 1 part mash parsnips, carrots or cauliflower to reduce the calories by nearly 75 per cent. Use a little light evaporated milk and forgo the butter. Omit or go easy on the gravy.
7. Potato pancakes (latkes), 2 pancakes	400	Use extra-virgin olive oil instead of higher-fat kinds such as corn oil, and toss out the egg yolks.
8. Creamed corn (250 g/9 oz)	184	Enjoy regular cooked sweetcorn kernels instead.
9. Traditional stuffing, large serving	640	Try wild rice as stuffing instead, and bake it separately. Cooked inside the turkey, the stuffing absorbs too much fat from the meat.

Food	Calories per Serving	The Leaner Eat
10. Roast goose	519	Stick with roast turkey.
11. Prime rib	569 to 854, depending on the size of the slab	Control your portion size!
12. Roast pork with pineapple	466	Roast a pork fillet in the oven by removing the skin, draining the fat, and adding broth, fruit or bitter orange or orange juice instead of oil to keep it moist. Serve with pineapple canned in its own juice.
13. Tamales, 3	459	Rather than using fat or shortening, make the tamales with a healthier vegetable oil, such as olive or rapeseed. You can also save fat and calories by making them vegetarian with a Mexican cheese or Monterey Jack and adding a green chilli (jala-peño or Anaheim, for example) for an extra kick.
14. Lasagne, beef, 1 portion	377	Prepare vegetable lasagne and enjoy one portion instead of two. Or make lasagne the American way with lean beef mince, part-skimmed mozzarella, and low-fat ricotta cheese and omit the cream.
15. Pecan pie, 1 slice (⅛ of the 23 cm/ 9 in diameter pie)	503	Pumpkin pie is a better bet. Some weigh in at only 150 calories a slice.
16. Apple pie, 1 slice (⅛ of the 23 cm/ 9 in diameter pie)	411	Go for pumpkin pie instead.
17. Mince pies	200	It's okay if you eat one, but who can stop at one?

DOCTOR, CAN YOU PLEASE TELL ME

I love Christmas, but I dread it too, because when I start eating sweets, I can't stop. Why?

Sweet foods really do make you hungry. The more sweets you eat (no matter what kind), the more you crave them. Why? When you eat sugary stuff, your blood sugar (glucose) surges. Insulin then works hard to bring it down, and fast. But the plummet in blood glucose then increases your appetite. This may be why after you eat sweets you want more and more. Sweets also increase the feel-good brain chemical serotonin.

You've just got to cut back or avoid them altogether, and the cravings will ease up and may even disappear. Put off going grocery shopping for a while. The fattening stuff in your fridge will disappear first. After a few days the biscuits, the ice cream and mince pies are history. All that's left are the raw vegetables. This can force you to eat a healthy diet. If you procrastinate long enough before going shopping, you might have to end up eating a raw beetroot. My point is: out of sight, out of mind. If seasonal treats are calling your name, keep them out of reach – which means out of your house.

GET SKINNY SHORTCUT

No Sweets

from your sweetie. Chocolate may be dandy for romance, but it can mean love handles in a hurry. Just about everyone likes chocolates on Valentine's Day, but most people are not aware of its calories. Most small pieces of chocolate – those about 30 g (1 oz) or so – contain about 150 calories each. It's not uncommon for a box of chocolates to contain 10,000 calories or more. If you eat the whole box, those excess calories can pile up faster than empty sweet wrappers. And as far as timing goes, Valentine's Day is not calendar friendly, either. Most people are still trying to get rid of the excess weight they put on during Christmas and New Year. Ask your sweetie to romance you with flowers, perfume or a special spa day.

12

The 17 Day Diet
on the Road

●●●●●●●●●●●●●●●●●●

Ionce had a patient – I'll call her Tina – who flew occasionally. She was about 175 cm (5 ft 9 in) and weighed 70 kg (11 stone) – not too bad for her height.

Then she accepted a job that immediately put her on a lot of aeroplanes. Tina liked to travel. But whilst away from home she wasn't exercising or eating as she knew she should be, and the end result was that she gained 2.25 kg (5 lb) in the first year. Didn't seem like much. But the next year she did the same, and the next. Tina gained an average of 2.25 kg (5 lb) a year for five years. One look in the mirror told her even more graphically than her bathroom scales that she had an 'excess baggage' problem.

Tina wasn't about to quit her job, but she was determined to lose that extra 11 kg (25 lb). She succeeded. And she kept it off. Not only did she feel better, but the mirror told her that she looked better too. And according to the latest medical statistics, she should live longer as well. The only downside was that she had to buy all new clothes!

For Tina, losing that weight required a long-term commitment and a lot of determination. But she did it, even though she continues flying 160,000 km (100,000 miles) a year and dealing with all the stuff that goes along with that level of travel.

If you're a 'road warrior' like Tina, this chapter is for you. I've got some advice that I'm convinced will work for you as you take off weight whilst occupying the friendly skies, and elsewhere on your travels.

At the Airport

Let's be honest: most airport eateries aren't noted for the variety or quality of their offerings. Airports are filled with high-fat, high-sugar snacks. If I must chew on something, I stroll right past the kiosks selling junk food and look for places where I can buy fruit, low-fat yoghurt or a salad.

Carefully examine the menu in airport restaurants. You can usually find a low-fat or low-calorie selection. If you have to grab airport food, look for a way to bulk up your fibre intake with things like fresh fruit (especially berries), salads, whole grains and vegetable soups.

What if you can't find anything that qualifies as 'healthy'? Sometimes I simply go hungry for a bit longer. If I must order a less-than-healthy item, I eat only a small portion of it. (Be warned: this tactic requires extraordinary willpower.)

Be active. Avoid the moving walkway. Unless you're absolutely going to miss a connecting flight, walk briskly to your next gate using your own two feet without the mechanical help.

Walk the concourse. If you have time between connecting flights, start walking around at a comfortably fast pace. Sure, I know you might be tired after a long flight and don't want to trudge through the airport, pulling your suitcase through throngs of other passengers. But trust me, a little walk will rejuvenate you and prevent travel weight piling on. Try to get in at least 10 to 20 minutes of brisk walking.

On the Plane

Airline food is almost universally considered a bad dining experience. We've all seen those UFOs (unidentified fried objects) and had that ubiquitous chicken breast that has circumnavigated the globe many times by now. If you're on a flight that offers a meal service (or you're fortunate enough to have upgraded to a class that provides an actual meal), make the same choices you would in a restaurant. Choose the low-calorie, low-fat, healthy selections, and eat sparingly of those carb-rich items such as rolls and puddings that aren't very healthy. Also, use only half the salad dressing you're given, and don't put butter on the roll. Ask if you can have some fresh fruit as a substitute for dessert. Little things add up fast.

Try to eat like you would at home. So if you don't tend to polish off a three-course meal with a giant ice cream sundae at home, don't eat one on the plane. I guarantee it's not going to be the best ice cream sundae you've ever had, so why spoil your diet on something mediocre?

Don't drink too many calories. When the drinks trolley rolls your way, ask for water, tomato juice or a calorie-free diet drink. Say no to alcohol and drinks with caffeine because they contribute to dehydration. The snacks available on flights aren't the greatest, so pass those up too. I suggest bringing your own healthy stuff to snack on: fresh fruits, cut-up veggies or one of my Power Cookies.

On long flights, move around from time to time. I don't mean roam the aisle and get in the flight attendants' way. Just stand up every half hour or so and stretch your legs, arms and other muscles.

This doesn't just burn a few calories; it may help prevent deep-vein thrombosis (DVT), a serious medical complication of long flights. If your legs are immobile for long periods, blood can gather in the lower limbs and form a clot in the veins found in the muscles. If the clot then travels to the heart, lungs or brain, it can be fatal. You're more at risk of a deep-vein thrombosis if you're elderly, obese, have conditions such as cancer or another acute medical illness, and if you have undergone surgery, or are pregnant, on birth control pills or hormone replacement therapy.

There are other preventive measures you can take if you're at risk. A 20- to 30-minute brisk walk around the terminal building will keep your circulation going over several hours. Stay hydrated too. Alcohol dehydrates you and makes you less mobile, increasing the risk of blood clots. Lots of airlines now offer exercise routines that you can do in your seat.

Travelling by Car

Don't forget your cool bag, and pack your own meals, including low-fat snacks. Choose 98 per cent fat-free lunch meats, fresh fruits and vegetables and water. Enjoy the trip by stopping at rest areas instead of fast food chains. When eating from fast food chains, choose wisely from the menu. Skip the chips and mayonnaise. Go for the salads.

Food at the Hotel

Arriving at your hotel late in the evening after a long day of travel can make room service or a late-night restaurant seem very, very appealing. Don't give in! You may be hungry, but skip the meal. Avoid late-night eating. Eating heavy foods shortly before going to bed is one of the worst things you can do to your waistline.

If you must have something to eat, many hotels place a basket of apples at the front desk. Pick up one or two when you check in, and eat them instead.

Sticking to a healthy nutritional regime can be a challenge when you're away from home. No matter where you go, much of your enjoyment will likely include great meals in different destinations. Fortunately, there are ways to enjoy the local fare without the anxiety that can come from overeating.

Go online and research restaurants at your destination to determine which ones offer healthy choices. This exercise should be easy to carry out since many establishments pride themselves on their specialities, from fresh seafood, to barbecues, to ethnic dishes. If you're heading to a major tourist town, look for guidebooks listing eateries according to cuisine type, as well as price range.

Make a list of your leading picks in the following categories: best breakfasts, top lunch spots and healthy restaurants for dinner. Tuck it into your handbag, briefcase or glove compartment to keep it handy, so you'll have flexibility and enough choices for each category. When composing your list, ignore all-you-can-eat places.

Start Your Day Healthy

If you begin your day with smart choices, chances are you'll continue with the same mindset throughout the day. Cereal with semi-skimmed or skimmed milk, fruit, yoghurt, juice, bagels and the like are excellent choices. If you're staying in a hotel that offers complimentary breakfast or a free buffet, steer clear or limit your intake of greasy or fried items. Have regular, light meals throughout the day to keep your energy level up and calorie count in check. Of course, it's equally important to stay hydrated. Keep bottles of water to hand to prevent thirst and to curb hunger.

LEAN 17: 17 Packable, Travel-Worthy Snacks

1. 115 g/4 oz apple puree pots (unsweetened)

2. Fat-free pudding snack pots

3. 115 g/4 oz fruit pots, packed in fruit juice

4. Apple or pear

5. Muesli or organic granola

6. My *Power Cookie*

7. Cut up raw veggies: carrots, celery, sugar snap peas, pepper or cucumber strips

8. Baby carrots

9. Single-serving box of high-fibre cereal

10. String cheese

11. One hard-boiled egg

12. Small bag of fat-free popcorn

13. Small bag of grapes

14. Healthy sandwich with veggies

15. Beef or turkey jerky

16. Orange

17. Edamame

Exercising on the Road

Book a hotel with an exercise room, preferably one that's open 24 hours a day. This has become a 'must have' for me. These days, the only way I'll stay in a hotel that doesn't offer exercise facilities is if I'm forced into it (for example, if I have to stay at a specific hotel in connection with a medical convention or meeting I'm attending).

If the hotel doesn't have fitness equipment, it may be affiliated with a local gym where you can get a one-day pass for a small fee. Once you get there, try a new class. You might be surprised at how fun it can be to do something different in another city. You might be able to find yoga, indoor cycling or step classes.

Spend a minimum of 30 minutes a day (or night) on the treadmill or stationary bike. You'll be surprised how good you feel at the end of your exercise time. You'll be more clear-headed and energetic for your business meetings, too.

I like to exercise in the morning. That way, I get it over with. At the end of a travel day there are too many variables that may get in the way. Besides, if you work out in the morning, you'll perform better all day.

Be creative. Most hotel rooms have enough floor space to allow you to turn your room into a mini-gym. Pack workout DVDs or skipping ropes. Stack phone books for a step workout performed to a favourite exercise video.

Bring elastic exercise bands. Learn basic exercises by asking for help from a body-sculpting group exercise instructor or a personal trainer before you leave town. Practise so you can do the exercises proficiently whilst travelling. When you're back home the bands will come in handy when you want to work out in your house, or you can't make it to a health club.

But don't forget bodyweight exercises such press-ups, squats with some luggage in hand to add extra resistance and overhead presses with the phone book. Sit-ups, with or without luggage resting on your chest, and crunches, help round out any on-the-road fitness programme. If you travel light, tune into exercise programmes on television and join right in.

Mix business and pleasure. Go dancing at a local club. It's an easy way to burn calories and check out the local scene.

And don't forget your bathing costume. If the hotel has an on-site pool, swimming laps is a great way to work up a sweat (yes, you sweat whilst you swim) and wash away the day's stress.

Another trick I like is to ask for a room on the second floor or higher, so you can use the stairs in the hotel for a great workout. Mark off 17 minutes on your watch. Walk down the hall of the hotel to the stairs. Walk up a floor, then down the hallway of that floor. Go up another floor and walk that hall-way. Continue in this manner for 8½ minutes; then repeat the 'course' down and back to your room. Just make sure you get back to the right floor and the right room. I've made that mistake before. It's not a pretty picture, trying to get in a room that's not yours.

Also, I bypass the lift even if I'm carrying luggage and my room is located on the 12th floor. It's amazing how much cardiovascular benefit you can get from using the stairs instead of the lift as you come and go. Sometimes taking the stairs will get you to your room faster than the lift will.

If stairs aren't your thing, consider the outdoors. How about seeing sights by walking or riding a rented bicycle? When renting bicycles, rent helmets as well. Ask the local bicycle shop about the best and safest routes and for descriptions of the terrain (flat or hilly). Walking is a wonderful way to combine exploring a new place with maintaining fitness. It's my favourite travel workout because it lets me take in the local sights, smells and sounds. Wear supportive and comfortable shoes. Ask the hotel concierge for suggestions. Walking to your destination can also reduce taxi fares.

Whew. I think I just burnt 1000 calories writing about all that.

So many people tell me they can't stay fit whilst travelling, but I don't buy it – that just means they don't want it badly enough. Good planning helps you fit fitness into your travel plans.

Review:

* Make healthy choices at airports or on planes.

* Use the airport as a 'gym' if you have time. Walk the concourse for exercise.

* Choose wisely at hotels and when dining out.

* Start your day healthy with a nutritious breakfast and exercise.

* Book a hotel with a fitness centre, or turn your hotel room into a gym.

* Handle holidays by keeping up your exercise programme, planning for special dietary needs, focusing on non-food aspects of the holiday and making healthy choices.

How to Handle Holidays

'Would you like soup and salad to go with your meal?'

'What would you like for dessert?'

'Where should we eat today?'

'Let's try the midnight buffet.'

Recently, I was bombarded with these questions whilst on holiday. I was being offered 12-course meals, all-you-can-eat breakfast and lunch buffets and a grill that was open 24 hours a day.

But after days and days of enjoying delicious foods, I realised that holidays do not mean diet disaster. Holidays mean enjoying yourself whilst maintaining your weight. Yes, they present additional challenges when you are trying to lose weight and maintain an exercise programme. An example I hear over and over again from people is: 'I love going on cruises, but every time I do, I end up triggering myself to fall off my programme for the rest of the year.'

In cases like this what should you do? I'd never suggest that you stop going on cruises, all-inclusive holidays or other destinations where food is so prevalent. But I might propose that you look for ways to be more active on one of these holidays, or plan to make healthier food choices or replace one of your yearly holidays with another type of holiday that is more active.

Holidays are not incompatible with watching your diet. They can always fit right into your lifestyle, and you don't have to feel burdened every time you go for a weekend break or enjoy a holiday. There are always alternatives. Here are some practical suggestions to help you through holidays without undoing all the hard work you have put into losing weight:

- Decide on your goal over the holiday. Do you want to maintain your current weight or continue to keep losing weight? For weight loss you'll have to monitor your calorie intake; if maintaining your weight is your goal, then you can adjust your calories upwards slightly.

- If you have special dietary needs, plan accordingly. Some cruise lines, for example, offer healthy meals low in fat and sodium and allow special orders.

- Focus on the other enjoyable aspects of the holiday rather than the food – the locale, the sightseeing and the activities.

- Make healthy food choices as often as possible, with an emphasis on fruits, vegetables, whole grains and lean proteins. To keep your hunger in check, lean towards high-fibre foods and foods with a high water content, such as raw or steamed whole vegetables and fruits. A sensible approach can help you avoid overeating.

- Ask for special requests for food that may not be on the menu. Many resorts offer these types of dietary accommodations.

- Keep an eye on your serving sizes and always practise portion control.

- Join the walking, aerobics and dancing programmes when you're on a cruise or at a resort, and use the exercise equipment in the gym. Take the most active shore excursions, or visit ports of call on your own and use guidebooks to create your own walking tour.

- Sightseeing activities get the muscles moving, but choose a tour that allows you opportunities to exercise. For example, time on your own in a city means you can jog or take a vigorous walk to attractions and shops. Ask whether the lodgings on a tour have lap pools or exercise rooms. If you happen to splurge, get back on course straight away, whether this means taking a short walk or eating one healthy meal. Congratulate yourself for getting back on your programme and acting in a healthy manner. After a few times of doing this you'll develop a positive mindset and begin to believe you can accomplish whatever it is you want.

13

Shift Work on
the 17 Day Diet

I'm sure you've heard the song '9 to 5'. It has catchy lyrics, but they don't describe the real-life experience of about 3.6 million British people. That's how many shift workers – on duty evenings, nights or in some rotating or otherwise irregular schedule – the The Labour Force Survey of Spring 1997 found working in a shift pattern, about 14 per cent of the working population. And you may be one of them. Occupations affected include: the military, food services, transportation, manufacturing and industry, police, firefighters, security personnel and health-care providers.

Unlike nocturnal animals such as owls and mice, most humans have some trouble adjusting to this strange lifestyle of working at night and sleeping in the day. This is because shift work, including night work, disrupts the body's 'circadian rhythm' – the internal clock that governs eating, sleeping, body temperature and other regular biological processes, all hardwired and regulated to the rising and setting of the sun.

As it turns out, messing around with that clock can have some serious consequences for your weight. Shift workers have a higher prevalence of being overweight – a fact substantiated by research. There are four main reasons why.

First, regular eating and exercise habits are tough to maintain on shift work. You can get bored easily, so you tend to nibble on junk food in response. According to a study by the New York Obesity Research Center and published in *Nutrition* in 2000, late-shift workers gained an average of 4.3 kg (9½ lb) during their late-shift tenure, whilst their day-shift counterparts gained only 900 g (2 lb).

Second, there's a hormonal issue. When you sleep and eat at irregular times, your metabolism gets thrown out of whack. At night, during sleep, your body's insulin-making processes naturally go into hibernation. You're not eating so the body doesn't require much insulin to process glucose from food. But if you eat on your night shift, there's not much insulin action so your body drives nutrients toward fat accumulation this late in the day.

Third, digestive problems are at fault. Shift workers have two to three times as many digestive problems as their day-shift peers. During night time, your digestive system shuts down and doesn't secrete the normal enzymes. Plus your metabolism slows down in the evening. Many shift workers report diarrhoea or constipation, gastric and peptic ulcers, gastritis, nausea and weight gain.

Finally, there are sleep problems. Shift workers are amongst the most sleep-deprived segments of our population. It's tough to sleep soundly during the day, when your body clock is screaming for you to be up and about. Also, sleep deprivation drives down leptin, a hormone produced in fat cells that tells your brain when you're full. At the same time, your substandard snoozing causes a rise in ghrelin, a hormone that makes you feel like you haven't eaten since two Mondays ago. Numerous studies showed that those who sleep less than eight hours a night have lower levels of leptin, higher levels of ghrelin and more body fat than the long-slumbering subjects. Chronic sleep deprivation can thus drastically increase your risk of gaining weight.

The weird hours you keep as a shift worker have a bunch of nutritional land mines – so here are some ways to avoid diet traps, stay true to the 17 Day Diet, keep your body in top form and still get your job done.

Avoid Junk Food

One of the things you can do to improve your energy and overall health is to eat a healthy diet rich in vitamins and minerals. Those chocolate bars and packets of crisps in the vending machines at work may be tempting, but they're probably doing you more harm than good, reducing your energy levels and stamina even further. Doughnuts and cakes may give you an instant 'buzz', but the downside is that you'll crash, and large amounts of refined sugar can lead to extreme mood swings.

The same goes for drinks. Cut down on the cans of cola and other fizzy drinks (even the 'diet' variety) and avoid drinks with caffeine because you'll find it harder to sleep when you get home. Instead, go for water. It's important to keep hydrated, since dehydration can lead to headaches and fatigue.

On night shift eat small, light meals with lots of raw salads, fruits and veggies, as recommended on the 17 Day Diet. These will give you energy but won't make you sleepy.

Sometimes shifts are long, so if you take sandwiches, make them wholegrain bread. Try gluten-free bread. The older you get, the more difficult gluten is to digest and it can block the bowel. A healthy bowel that is moving will give you more energy.

Follow My Sample Shift Menus

Let's put these suggestions in concrete form. All Cycles of the 17 Day Diet are adaptable to shift work. It just takes a little bit of planning. If possible, take meals at approximately the same time each day, either midday or early evening, irrespective of whether you are on night shift. Follow the guidelines below and you'll get in better sync, lose weight and be more alert.

Sample Shift Menu – Afternoon Shift
(Start time between 2.00 p.m. and 4.00 p.m.;
finish time between 10.00 p.m. and midnight)

Generally, if you work an afternoon shift, it's best to have your main meal (dinner) in the middle of the day rather than in the middle of your shift. You'll burn off your food better and stay more alert on your shift.

Here are some meal-planning suggestions for each Cycle.

Time of Day/Meal	Accelerate Cycle	Activate Cycle	Achieve Cycle	Arrive Cycle
8.00 to 10.00 a.m./ Breakfast	2 scrambled eggs, fresh fruit, 175 g/ 6 oz yoghurt	30 g/1oz porridge oats, cooked; 4 egg whites, scrambled; fresh fruit	55 g/2 oz high-fibre cereal; 240 ml/8 fl oz skimmed or soya milk or other substitute; fresh fruit	Stick to whole grains and protein

continued on the next page

Time of Day/Meal	Accelerate Cycle	Activate Cycle	Achieve Cycle	Arrive Cycle
1.00 to 2.00 p.m. Dinner (before shift)	Grilled chicken breast with liberal amounts of any vegetables, steamed or raw; fresh fruit	Grilled pork chops; steamed veggies; 70 g/ 2½ oz sweetcorn; 175 g/ 6 oz yoghurt or other probiotic serving; fresh fruit	Grilled chicken; steamed vegetables such as asparagus, runner beans, broccoli or cauliflower; fresh fruit	Focus on protein-rich foods to keep you alert
7.00 to 8.00 p.m. *Lunch at work break*	Tuna tossed with 1 tablespoon olive oil and a tablespoon of vinegar, served over a generous bed of lettuce; 175 g/6 oz yoghurt or other probiotic serving to help with digestion	Prawn salad: Cooked prawns, 30 g/ 1 oz chopped onion, generous bed of lettuce leaves, 1 tomato (large) and 1 tablespoon olive oil; 175 g/6 oz yoghurt or other probiotic serving to help with digestion	Pitta sandwich: 1 whole grain pitta filled with chopped lettuce and tomato; 20 g/ ¾ oz crumbled fat-free feta cheese; 1 tablespoon Italian salad dressing; 10 baby carrots; 175 g/ 6 oz yogurt or other probiotic serving to help with digestion	Continue focusing on protein-rich foods. Munch on fresh fruit and vegetables. Don't overload yourself on carbs. Be sure to include probiotic foods to help with digestion.
After work/ before bedtime	Fresh fruit	Have a carb or two; bananas are a good choice as they help with sleep	Have a carb or two; bananas are a good choice as they help with sleep	Have a carb or two; bananas are a good choice as they help with sleep

Sample Shift Menu – Night Shift
(midnight to 8.00 a.m.)

Generally, night shift workers should snack lightly during their shift, eat a moderate breakfast and have dinner before their shift starts.

Here's a look at how to plan your diet.

Time of Day/Meal	Accelerate Cycle	Activate Cycle	Achieve Cycle	Arrive Cycle
When you wake up	2 scrambled eggs, fresh fruit, 175 g/ 6 oz yoghurt	30 g/1 oz porridge oats, cooked; 4 egg whites, scrambled; fresh fruit	55 g/2 oz high-fibre cereal; 240 ml/8 fl oz semi-skimmed, skimmed or soya milk or other dairy substitute; fresh fruit	Egg-white omelette with spinach; one slice of brown toast with jam; 85 g/ 3 oz of fresh strawberries; tea, coffee or water
6.00 to 8.00 p.m./ Dinner (before shift)	Grilled chicken breast with liberal amounts of any vegetables, steamed or raw; fresh fruit	Grilled pork chops; steamed veggies; 70 g/2½ oz sweetcorn	Grilled chicken; steamed vegetables such as asparagus, runner beans, broccoli or cauliflower; fresh fruit	Dinner: Green salad with sliced tomato, oil and vinegar dressing; ½ grilled chicken breast with lemon and herbs; 100 g/3½ oz of brown rice; steamed broccoli; fresh fruit; soda water with lemon or water

continued on the next page

Time of Day/Meal	Accelerate Cycle	Activate Cycle	Achieve Cycle	Arrive Cycle
3.00 to 4.00 a.m. **Lunch at work break**	Tuna tossed with 1 tablespoon olive oil and a tablespoon of vinegar, served over a generous bed of lettuce; 175 g/6 oz yoghurt or other probiotic serving to help with digestion	Prawn salad: Cooked prawns, 30 g/1 oz chopped onion, generous bed of lettuce leaves, 1 tomato (large), and 1 tablespoon olive oil; 175 g/6 oz yoghurt or other probiotic serving to help with digestion	Pitta sandwich: 1 whole grain pitta filled with chopped lettuce and tomato; 20 g/¾ oz crumbled fat-free feta cheese; 1 tablespoon Italian salad dressing; 10 baby carrots; 175 g/6 oz yoghurt or other probiotic serving to help with digestion	Tossed green salad with avocado and 115 g/4 oz of steamed salmon, oil and vinegar dressing; soda water with lemon or water; 175 g/6 oz yoghurt or other probiotic serving to help with digestion
After shift, before sleep	Fresh fruit	Have a carb or two; bananas are a good choice as they help with sleep	Have a carb or two; bananas are a good choice as they help with sleep	Have a carb or two; bananas are a good choice as they help with sleep

LEAN 17: 17 Foods that Keep You Alert

Most of the foods on the 17 Day Diet can help you stay more alert and are perfect for shift work. Choose more of the following foods to add to your diet if you're a shift worker.

Food	Alertness Factor
1. Beef, extra lean	High in iron, a mineral that improves memory, alertness and attention span.

Food	Alertness Factor
2. Beetroots	Contains phenylalanine, an amino acid that helps relay signals from one brain cell to another.
3. Blueberries	Excellent source of antioxidants and 'anthocyanins', compounds thought to help protect brain cells from toxins – improves use of glucose in the brain and promotes communication between brain cells.
4. Broccoli	Packed with antioxidants and phytonutrients that help protect brain tissue from toxins.
5. Carrots	High in beta-carotene and other natural substances that help protect brain tissue from toxins.
6. Chicken	High in tyrosine, an amino acid required for the production of the alertness chemicals dopamine, epinephrine and norepinephrine. When your brain is producing these, you think and react more quickly, and feel more motivated, attentive and mentally energetic.
7. Citrus fruits	Contain vitamin C and other antioxidants that help maintain sharp memory and help brain cells resist damage.
8. Edamame	Contains phenylalanine, an amino acid that helps relay signals from one brain cell to another.
9. Eggs	High in the B vitamin choline, which helps with memory.
10. Egg whites	High in protein, which can improve alertness by increasing levels of norepinephrine, which helps keep your brain at its sharpest.
11. Hot chillies	Contain the fiery-tasting chemical capsaicin. Capsaicin stimulates circulation, aids digestion, opens your nasal passages and, even better, sends a feeling of euphoria straight to your brain.
12. Pulses	Provide glucose to fuel the brain, and the fibre they contain slows the absorption of glucose, helping to maintain stable levels of energy and support alertness and concentration over time.

continued on the next page

Food	Alertness Factor
13. Pork	Loaded with vitamin B1, which protects myelin, a fatty substance that helps facilitate communication amongst cells.
14. Cos lettuce	High in folate, a B vitamin important for memory and nerve cell health.
15. Spinach	Packed with iron, which is involved memory, concentration, and mental functioning.
16. Tuna	Full of omega-3 fatty acids, which help build and maintain myelin.
17. Yoghurt	A probiotic food that has been found in many studies to boost mental alertness. Yoghurt and other probiotic foods are great foods for night shift work, as they help digestion.

The Exercise Connection

Let's look on the bright side of the night shift: you get to go to the gym whilst almost everybody else is at work. Try picking a good time early in your 'day'. Even if you do only half your usual workout, you'll be moving your body, and you'll feel better. Seventeen minutes of exercise at least three times each week (though not just before bedtime) will help reduce stress and feelings of fatigue and increase your sense of well-being.

Be consistent with your training and add in some fun cross-training activities. You might have more time for outdoor bicycle rides, for example, with your night-shift schedule. As you catch up on your sleep, train longer and/or harder until you're back to your former training level.

Sleep Sense

Working when everyone else is asleep has advantages: less traffic for commuters, seeing newspapers being delivered, being around when the children get home from school and maybe even a better pay rate. But getting enough rest isn't one of them.

Night-shift workers typically don't get the seven to eight hours of sleep the vast majority of people need, and that's dangerous for your health, your weight and for other people on the road when you're yawning behind the wheel.

NOT THE USUAL 9 TO 5: Other Health Effects of Shift Work

Conditions	Reason	Strategies
Cardiovascular	Shift workers have more adverse lifestyle behaviours such as higher tendency to smoke, not exercise and eat junk food – all of which hurt the heart. In one study 665 day workers were compared with 659 shift workers. The late-night workers had twice the risk of low HDL cholesterol, 40% higher risk of high triglycerides and 19% higher risk of abdominal adiposity.	• Stop smoking • Exercise • Eat nutritiously
Breast Cancer	The risk may be associated with exposure to light during the night, when you should be sleeping. The hormone melatonin may play a role. Production of the hormone, which usually occurs during the 'dark' period of a person's day, is disrupted by light exposure. The resulting dearth of melatonin may allow very small colonies of existing cancerous cells to flourish.	• Don't take melatonin, unless specifically recommended by a doctor. Whilst you'd think it would be helpful, it can actually throw a spanner into the smooth functioning of the circadian system and worsen the disruption to your biological clock.
Diabetes	Shift work can disrupt the body's insulin-making processes, potentially causing insulin resistance. With insulin resistance, the body doesn't use insulin properly. Glucose gets locked out of cells, and it clutters up the bloodstream.	• Have regular check-ups to monitor changes in blood sugar. • Avoid refined carbohydrates such as sweets, white bread and baked goods. • Exercise on a regular basis to help the body better regulate blood sugar.

Sleeping during the day tends to be less restful too, so no wonder one in five night workers reports falling asleep on the job. I can't give you a surefire recipe for sound sleep during the day, but I have several techniques that should help. Even if each technique helps you sleep only a little better, all together they may let you get the rest you deserve and need.

One key strategy is to maintain a somewhat constant schedule. Don't sleep from noon to 8.00 p.m. on Friday, then try sleeping nights on Saturday and Sunday, then switch back to day sleeping on Monday. Even if you alter your schedule a little, don't change too much. A study in the *New Zealand Journal of Psychology* advises a strategy called 'anchor sleep', in which you include a three- to four-hour block of sleep time on non-shift-work days that coincides with your anticipated sleep time on shift-work days.

Sleep as soon as possible after the night shift. If you delay sleep after the night shift, your body will begin to warm up and prepare for the day's activity.

Change your lights. You want the period whilst you're sleeping – whether you're a night-shift or a daytime worker – to be as dark as possible. Consider blackout curtains, a sleep mask or anything else that reduces light. This is vital, as melatonin, the hormone of sleep that increases drowsiness, is suppressed by daylight even through closed eyelids. Light passes through your eyes and sets your brain's internal clock. You want to trick your brain into believing that day is night, and vice versa. No light? It must be night.

No matter what your shift, you may want to consider installing a low-wattage red bulb in the bathroom so that when you get up in the middle of your sleep cycle, it isn't disturbed by the shock of bright lights.

Sleep in a quiet part of the house, away from traffic noise and household activity. Tell family and friends about your schedule and ask them to call you only during waking hours. Give them a copy of your shift schedule.

Regulate your use of caffeine. Many of us toss back coffee to keep up energy at work. Not a good idea. It's tempting for night workers to use caffeine at the end of their shifts because it's when they're most sluggish, but that's only likely to continue to chip away at sleep quality.

Eat a banana or drink some warm milk before going to bed. Both these foods contain l-tryptophan, an amino acid known to be a natural sleep inducer. L-tryptophan releases serotonin, a sleep-inducing brain chemical.

Avoid alcohol prior to sleep. It is a diuretic and interferes with the quality of sleep. Try a herbal tea instead. Teas containing valerian root can be a safe, effective way to sleep when you really need to. As with any sleep aid, it should be used sparingly, however. Some people feel groggy upon awakening if they've taken valerian. (The best sleep aid is regular exercise.)

If you're a shift worker, you have to take extra care of yourself. It's worth your quality of life and livelihood to do so.

Review:

* Shift workers suffer from obesity and other illnesses more often than people who work regular hours.

* If you're a shift worker, avoid junk food. Have your main meal in the middle of the day if you work an afternoon shift, and have dinner just before your shift starts if you work the midnight shift.

* Punctuate your night with natural foods that keep you alert.

* Maintain a consistent exercise schedule.

* Practise good sleep health: keep your bedroom as dark as possible, sleep in a quiet part of your house, limit your use of caffeine and alcohol, and have a snack such as a banana and some warm milk prior to going to bed.

* Talk to your family doctor if you think you might be suffering from shift work disorder, see below.

CHECK-UP: Do You Have Shift Work Disorder?

The term shift work disorder, or SWD, may be new to you. But if you have a non-traditional work schedule, or work shifts, and are often tired on the job or have trouble sleeping, it's a condition you should learn more about.

Shift work disorder is a recognised medical condition that can be diagnosed and treated by a doctor. It occurs when your body's internal clock, or circadian rhythm, is out of sync with your work schedule.

Many people who work outside the traditional 9-to-5 schedule need to be awake when the body's natural cycle calls for sleep. This disturbance of the circadian rhythm can lead to excessive sleepiness during waking hours or trouble sleeping during sleeping hours. If you're a shift worker, take the following quiz to see if you might have shift work disorder. Circle either 'yes' or 'no'.

continued on the next page

1. Do you feel tired no matter how much sleep you try to get?   **Yes   No**

2. Are you often less alert than you could be?   **Yes   No**

3. Do you have difficulty falling asleep or staying asleep?   **Yes   No**

4. Are you unaware of your total sleeping hours per day?   **Yes   No**

5. Have you been making more errors at work than usual due to lack of focus and general sense of fatigue?   **Yes   No**

6. Do you frequently suffer from heartburn or indigestion?   **Yes   No**

7. Do you experience occasional morning headaches?   **Yes   No**

8. Has your work, home or social life been negatively affected by sleeping problems?   **Yes   No**

9. Have you been experiencing unexplained weight gain?   **Yes   No**

10. Have you been experiencing irregular menstrual cycles?   **Yes   No**

11. Do you fall asleep whilst driving, in meetings, whilst reading a book or whilst watching television?   **Yes   No**

Scoring: If you answer yes to three or more of these questions, you may be dealing with shift work disorder. Consult your doctor. He or she can help manage your symptoms. Only a change in shift work can resolve SWD, but there are some things you can do to try to cope with your symptoms, and they bear repeating:

- Avoid alcohol and other substances before bedtime
- Get a full eight hours of sleep each day
- Turning on bright lights may help diminish drowsiness when you need to be awake
- Eliminate noise and light from your sleep area
- Try to stick to your sleep and wake schedule, even on weekends

14

The 17 Day Diet
Recipes

One healthy practice that will make a big difference in your weight loss is to cook your own food. Now before you start to panic, rest assured that you don't need to shout and jump and spin knives, or make meals that look like a major work of art. You need some easy recipes – that's all. I can help you with that.

This batch of recipes is easy to follow and simple to prepare. There are no long lists of ingredients, complicated cooking methods or hard-to-understand directions. All the recipes are built around the foods you eat on the 17 Day Diet.

They're are all low in fat and calories, made leaner and healthier by using cooking methods such as grilling, baking or lightly stir-frying. When the recipes do call for oil, it is always a healthy one such as olive oil.

Some of the recipes make just one serving. If others in your family are following the 17 Day Diet, you can easily prepare these single-serving recipes in extra quantities. Other recipes feature multiple servings. Any leftovers can be refrigerated or frozen. That way, you can defrost and/or reheat them in the micro-wave for a quick, healthy meal.

Once you get the hang of this way of cooking and eating, expect to lose your taste for greasy, sugary stuff. Why? Because tastes are learnt. Just as you learnt to like fattening, sugary or salty foods, your taste buds can be retrained to enjoy fresh, delicious and healthy dishes. For example, it's possible to retrain your taste buds by using herbs and spices. Salt-free seasoning blends are a good way to help yourself get out of the habit of sprinkling salt on everything. Your taste buds do adapt to what you eat.

I encourage you to get creative beyond these recipes. Most of us use the same ten to 12 recipes most of the time. Why not try tweaking them to fit the 17 Day Diet? Here are some suggestions:

- **Dairy Products.** If a recipe calls for dairy products, you can always use low-fat and occasionally fat-free substitutions. For example, if a recipe uses 225 g (8 oz) of regular soured cream, you can usually substitute fat-free natural yoghurt (Greek-style yoghurt is ideal), or blended low-fat cottage cheese. Yoghurt or silken tofu can be mixed with low-fat mayonnaise in dishes such as coleslaw, tuna and chicken salads.

- **Meats.** When selecting meat minces, look for those 90 per cent fat-free or higher. These are generally more expensive per kilogramme, but you are getting more meat for your money because less fat is incorporated in the total product. If you cook meat mince, drain away excess fat after browning it. Simply place kitchen paper in a colander and pour the browned meat in so the paper can absorb the fat. If a recipe calls for a high-fat meat such as bacon, you can reduce the fat by 50 to 60 per cent by using a smaller amount of chopped bacon to impart the flavour. Or try using lean back bacon instead.

- **Bad Fats.** You can reduce or eliminate fats in recipes. For example, when sautéing or frying, simply coat non-stick pans with a spritz of vegetable oil cooking spray (0 calories) rather than using vegetable fat or butter.

- **Spice it up.** Get in the habit of using high-flavour ingredients such as fresh herbs, zesty spices and seasonal fruits to invigorate dishes, rather than fat or oil. Another tip: buy an oil mister at a specialist kitchen shop. Simply pour oil such as linseed or olive oil into the spray bottle and then spray a fine mist of the oil over the pan or the food. This process cuts the amount of oil that you use drastically and cuts calories from fat.

- **Desserts.** Fruit makes a great dessert, but by itself may be boring to eat. Try dressing up a bowl of strawberries with a drizzle of sugar-free chocolate syrup. Also, you can easily redesign your favourite pudding recipes to use less sugar, fat and calories by switching to lower-fat ingredients and learning how to cook with a natural low-calorie sweetener.

• **Salt.** Are you watching your sodium intake? If so, start by using half the amount called for in the recipe. Continue to reduce the amount until you find the minimum amount needed to season the recipe. Or replace the salt with lemon or lime juice, flavoured vinegar, fresh onion or garlic, onion or garlic powder, pepper, chilli powder, ginger or herb-only seasonings. Use low-sodium soy sauce or hot mustard sauce to replace regular soy sauce. Season food with spices and herbs as an alternative to adding salt.

Now – the 17 Day Diet recipes. Enjoy!

Dr Mike's Power Cookie

Ingredients

70 g/2½ oz unsweetened apple purée

2 tablespoons almond paste

1 tablespoon linseed oil

10 packets of natural low-calorie sweetener

4 tablespoons agave nectar

1 medium egg

½ teaspoon vanilla extract

85 g/3 oz wholemeal flour

½ teaspoon bicarbonate of soda

1 teaspoon cinnamon

½ teaspoon salt

¼ teaspoon black pepper

2 scoops vanilla whey protein powder

175 g/6 oz porridge oats

150 g/5 oz dried cherries

55 g/2 oz flaked almonds

Directions

Heat oven to Gas Mark 4/180°C/fan oven 160°C. Beat together apple purée, almond paste, linseed oil, natural sweetener and agave nectar. Beat in egg and vanilla. Mix well. Add flour, bicarbonate of soda, salt, pepper and whey powder. Beat thoroughly. Stir in oats, cherries and almonds. Mix well. Drop the batter by large tablespoons onto a baking sheet that has been sprayed with vegetable cooking spray. Divide dough so that you have 18 cookies. Flatten each cookie with the back of the spoon. Bake for 16 to 18 minutes or until brown. Remove from oven. Cool and store in a plastic container. Each cookie supplies 128 calories and can be enjoyed on the Activate, Achieve and Arrive Cycles for breakfast or as a snack. Each cookie counts as 1 protein and 1 natural starch.

Kefir Smoothie

Ingredients

240 ml/8 fl oz unsweetened kefir

115 g/4 oz unsweetened berries

1 tablespoon sugar-free fruit jam

or 1 tablespoon agave nectar

1 tablespoon linseed oil

Directions

Place all ingredients in a blender and blend until smooth. Makes 1 large serving.

Yoghurt Fruitshake

Ingredients

120 ml/4 fl oz kefir

85 g/3 oz sugar-free fruit-flavoured yoghurt

115 g/4 oz unsweetened berries

Directions

Place all ingredients in a blender and blend until smooth. Makes 1 large serving.

Egg-White Veggie Frittata

Ingredients

4 egg whites, beaten

1 plum tomato, chopped

Fresh spinach, handful

Salt and pepper, to taste

Directions

Coat a small frying plan with vegetable oil cooking spray. Add beaten egg whites. Stir in tomato and spinach. Cook on a medium-low heat until egg whites are cooked through. Lift from pan with a spatula, and season lightly as desired. Makes 2 servings

Spanish Omelette

Ingredients

1 egg

2 egg whites

⅛ teaspoon salt

⅛ teaspoon black pepper

1 tablespoon olive oil

45 g/1½ oz tomato, diced

20 g/¾ oz onion, diced

15 g/½ oz fat-free Cheddar cheese, grated

Directions

In a medium bowl, whisk together egg, egg whites, salt and black pepper. Heat a frying pan over a medium-high heat. Add olive oil and swirl pan to coat bottom and sides. Add beaten eggs and tilt pan to spread mixture across entire pan bottom. Cook for about 30 seconds. With a palette knife, gently lift sides of omelette and tilt pan to distribute more uncooked egg to the pan's surface. Once the egg begins to set, sprinkle the tomato, onion and Cheddar cheese over one side of the omelette. Carefully fold the other side of the omelette over the filling. Makes 1 serving.

Greek Egg Scramble

Ingredients

4 egg whites	20 g/¾ oz reduced-fat feta cheese, crumbled
115 g/4 oz red onions, chopped	⅛ teaspoon salt
45 g/1½ oz tomato, diced	⅛ teaspoon black pepper

Directions

In a medium bowl, whisk together all ingredients. Pour into a small frying pan that has been coated with vegetable oil cooking spray. Cook over a medium-low heat until eggs are cooked through. Makes 1 serving.

Niçoise Salad

Ingredients

85 g/3 oz canned light tuna	1 small tomato, sliced
Cooked French beans, chilled (55–115 g/2–4 oz)	Lettuce (the darker, the better)
2 spring onions, chopped	1 tablespoon olive oil
	2 tablespoons balsamic vinegar

Directions

Place cooked French beans, spring onion and tomatoes on a liberal bed of lettuce. Top with tuna. Drizzle with the olive oil and balsamic vinegar and season lightly. Makes 1 serving.

Super Salad

Ingredients:

Lettuce, any variety

Cucumbers

Onions

Tomatoes

Any salad vegetable from the 17 Day Diet lists

2 hard-boiled eggs, chopped

2 tablespoons olive oil or linseed oil

60 ml/2 fl oz balsamic vinegar

Directions

Combine lettuce with salad veggies and hard-boiled eggs. Toss with olive oil or linseed oil and balsamic vinegar. Lightly season. Makes 1 serving.

Balsamic Artichoke

Ingredients

4 fresh globe artichokes

60 ml/2 fl oz balsamic vinegar

Fat-free salad dressing

Directions

Place artichokes in a large saucepan. Cover with water. Pour in balsamic vinegar. Cover and cook for about 1 hour on moderate heat or until artichokes are tender, including the stem. Let cool. Serve with fat-free salad dressing for dipping. Makes 4 servings.

Spinach Salad

Ingredients

Baby spinach leaves (these taste less bitter than regular spinach leaves)

Assortment of salad veggies (onions, cucumbers, tomatoes, etc.)

20 g/¾ oz reduced-fat feta cheese, crumbled

1 tablespoon olive or linseed oil

2 tablespoons balsamic vinegar

Directions

Place a large bed of baby spinach leaves on a plate. Top spinach leaves with salad veggies and feta cheese. Drizzle with olive or linseed oil mixed with the balsamic vinegar. Season to taste. Makes 1 serving.

Taco Salad

Ingredients

450 g/1 lb lean turkey mince

1 sachet of taco seasoning

Generous bed of lettuce

175 g/6 oz chopped tomatoes

400 g/14 oz chopped onions

Salsa

75 g/2½ oz reduced-fat Cheddar cheese, grated

Directions

In a saucepan, brown the turkey mince over a moderate heat. Add the taco seasoning and cook according to packet instructions. Place generous servings of lettuce on 4 plates. Top with turkey mixture, tomatoes, onions, salsa and cheese. Makes 4 servings.

Village Salad

Ingredients

2 tomatoes, chopped

½ teaspoon sea salt

40 g/1½ oz red onion, chopped

1 teaspoon dried oregano

1 tablespoon olive oil

20 g/¾ oz reduced-fat feta cheese, crumbled

Directions

Combine tomatoes with sea salt; let sit for 5 minutes. Then mix tomato and salt together with the rest of the ingredients. Makes 1 serving.

Lettuce Wraps

Ingredients

1 baked chicken breast, diced

1 spring onion, diced

85 g/3 oz red grapes, chopped

15 g/½ oz celery, chopped

1 tablespoon olive oil

Salt and pepper to taste

2 to 3 Little Gem or iceberg lettuce leaves

Directions

Mix together all ingredients except the lettuce. Refrigerate until chilled. To serve, take 1 lettuce leaf at a time, and spoon a heaped tablespoon of the chicken mixture into the centre. Wrap the lettuce around the filling. Makes 1 serving.

Spicy Yoghurt Dip and Veggies

Ingredients

900 g/2 lbs fat-free natural yoghurt
Garlic powder
Onion powder

Seasoned salt
Cut-up fresh veggies

Directions

Line a sieve with a coffee filter or white kitchen paper. Place the sieve over a bowl (this catches the liquid that will drain off the yoghurt). Spoon the yogurt in the filter-lined sieve. Cover and refrigerate for 8 hours or overnight. This process yields about 475 ml/16 fl oz of yoghurt cheese. Season the cheese lightly with the seasonings suggested above, or add freshly chopped herbs such as parsley, rosemary or thyme. 85 g/3 oz of yoghurt cheese = 1 probiotic serving. Use as dip for fresh vegetables.

Chicken-Vegetable Soup

Ingredients

4 baked chicken breasts, diced into
   small chunks
150 g/5 oz cabbage, chopped
1 large carrot, chopped
225 g/8 oz okra, sliced
1 large onion, chopped

2 large celery sticks with leaves, chopped
400 g/14 oz can of chopped tomatoes
400 ml/14 fl oz fat-free chicken broth
1½ teaspoons salt
¼ teaspoon pepper

Directions

Place all ingredients, except chicken, in a large pan and simmer for 1 hour or until vegetables are soft. Add chicken and heat thoroughly. Enjoy this soup for lunch or dinner. Makes 4 servings.

Marinated Vegetable Salad

Ingredients

4 large handfuls of raw vegetables
(French beans, cauliflower,
Brussels sprouts, artichoke hearts, etc.)
Fat-free Italian dressing

Lettuce
Bottled roasted red peppers

Directions

The night before, steam some raw vegetables over at least 475 ml/16 fl oz of water until they're tender but still crisp. Place in a glass dish and pour fat-free Italian dressing over veggies. Refrigerate overnight. Drain and serve on a bed of lettuce topped with roasted red peppers (no oil) from a bottle. Makes 2 to 4 servings.

Aubergine Parmesan

Ingredients

1 large aubergine, peeled

4 egg whites

Fat-free Parmesan cheese

Garlic powder, to taste

250 g/9 oz reduced-calorie pasta sauce

Directions

Preheat oven to Gas Mark 6/200°C/fan assist 180°C. Cut aubergine into 5 mm/ ¼ inch slices. In a shallow dish, beat egg whites and 4 tablespoons of water until foamy. Dip aubergine slices into egg whites, then into fat-free Parmesan cheese, pressing cheese into aubergine. Place aubergine on a prepared baking tray that has been sprayed with vegetable spray and sprinkle with garlic powder. Spray vegetable cooking spray over aubergine slices. Bake 30 minutes in pre-heated oven, turning aubergine over after 20 minutes, until golden brown and cooked through. Cover with low-cal pasta sauce. Bake for 20 minutes, or until aubergine is piping hot and sauce is bubbly. Makes 2 large servings.

Sesame Fish

Ingredients

450 g/1 lb of tilapia or other white fish

2 tablespoons olive oil

2 tablespoons rice vinegar

2 tablespoons light soy sauce

1 teaspoon chopped garlic

20 g/¾ oz sesame seeds

Vegetable oil spray

Directions

Spray a grill pan with vegetable oil spray to prevent fish from sticking. Place tilapia in the pan. Whisk together olive oil, rice vinegar, soy sauce and garlic until well blended. Pour over fish. Sprinkle sesame seeds over fish. Grill at medium heat for about 20 minutes or until fish flakes easily with a fork.

Makes 4 servings.

Salmon Lemonato

Ingredients

2 wild salmon fillets

1 tablespoon olive oil

3 lemons

1 teaspoon dried oregano

3 cloves fresh garlic, chopped

Vegetable oil cooking spray

Directions

Preheat oven to Gas Mark 4/180°C/fan assist 160°C. Place salmon in a shallow glass dish that has been sprayed with vegetable oil cooking spray. Drizzle olive oil over salmon. Top with garlic. Squeeze the juice of the lemons over the salmon and sprinkle with oregano. Bake for 25 minutes. Makes 2 servings.

Oven Barbecued Chicken

Ingredients

4 skinless boneless chicken breasts

80 ml/3 fl oz reduced-sugar tomato ketchup

2 tablespoons Worcestershire sauce

1 tablespoon agave nectar

1 teaspoon chilli powder

Vegetable oil cooking spray

Directions

Preheat oven to Gas Mark 4/180°C/fan assist 160°C. Place chicken breasts in a baking tin that has been sprayed with vegetable oil cooking spray. Bake for 20–25 minutes. In the meantime, stir together ketchup, Worcestershire sauce, agave nectar and chilli powder to make the barbecue sauce. Remove chicken breasts from oven and coat with sauce. Return to oven and bake for 10 more minutes. Makes 4 servings.

Turkey Black Bean Chilli

Ingredients

450 g/1 lb lean turkey mince

400 g/14 oz can black beans
   (For Cycles 2 and 3 only)

150 g/5 oz onion, chopped

500 g/18 oz passata

1 tablespoon chilli powder

1 teaspoon Kosher salt

½ teaspoon black pepper

Directions

In a saucepan, brown the turkey mince over a moderate heat. Add the remainder of the ingredients. Simmer for 20 minutes. Makes 4 servings.

Low-Carb Primavera Delight

Ingredients

1 spaghetti squash
   or 2 butternut squashes
200 g/7 oz fresh broccoli, chopped
1 small onion, diced

2 garlic cloves. diced
1 tablespoon olive oil

Directions

Spaghetti squash is a great substitute for pasta. To prepare it, cut it in half (lengthways). Scoop out the seeds and pulp as you would with any squash or pumpkin. Place it in a glass baking dish with about 1 cm/½ inch of water, rind side up. Bake for 40–45 minutes in a preheated oven at Gas Mark 5/190°C/fan assist 170°C. You can also microwave the squash for 8–10 minutes per half on high. Let the squash stand for a few minutes after baking or microwaving. Separate strands by running a fork through the flesh 'from stem to stern' direction. Place strands in a separate bowl.

In a medium frying pan, sauté broccoli, onion, garlic and oil until vegetables are crisp and tender. Add squash and heat thoroughly. Serve on plates topped with heated pasta sauce. Makes 4 servings.

Note: if you can't find spaghetti squash in a supermarket, it is easy to grow. Or you can susbstitute butternut squash, though you won't be able to separate it into strands to resemble spaghetti.

15

Doctor,
Can You Please Tell Me More?

∙ ∙

The **17 Day Diet** is simple, easy and do-able, but still questions arise from time to time. Here are the questions I'm frequently asked, along with my answers. This information will help you.

Diet Issues

Q. I just need to lose the 'last 4.5 kg (10 lb)'. How long should I stay on the diet?

A. You should lose those 4.5 kg (10 lb) rapidly on Cycle 1 if you follow it to the letter. Or you may have to continue into Cycle 2. It all depends on your individual metabolism. Everyone is different and loses weight at different rates. If you'd like to accelerate your weight loss and get to that goal faster, increase your exercise time and intensity each day. Just hang in there, don't get discouraged and you'll achieve your goal weight in no time.

Q. Can I switch some dinners to lunch, and lunch to dinners?

A. Yes, you may switch lunches with dinners. It is good idea to eat lightly in the evening anyway. I recommend switching lunches and dinners if you are a shift worker, especially. If you switch, be sure to not eat carbs past 2.00 p.m.

Q. Is the 17 Day Diet safe for everyone?

A. The diet is designed for people in normal health. Anyone who goes on this diet should have the blessing of his or her doctor. Do not follow this diet if you have type 1 diabetes, any serious medical disease or if you are pregnant or breast-feeding.

Q. I've got great results so far on Cycle 1. Can't I just stay on it?

A. Great job with your weight loss! That tells me you have a strong will for healthier habits and respect the gift of your health. Keep going! I don't advise staying on Cycle 1 for more than 17 days, however. The diet is carefully designed to keep your metabolism charged up, to prevent plateaus and to re-introduce foods gradually back into your life. It's best that you follow all three Cycles as described. Then after 51 days, you get to return to Cycle 1 for continued weight loss if necessary.

Q. Can I drink fruit-flavoured green tea on the diet?

A. Yes, as long as it is not sweetened with added sugar. Many green teas in the supermarket are flavoured with a hint of natural fruit and no added sugar. These are very tasty and can be enjoyed hot or cold.

Q. When you say 'liberal amounts' of a food, does that mean a huge piece of meat or second helpings of those foods?

A. No. It's important to not overload your stomach. Use my Hunger/Fullness Meter to keep that from happening. Eat until satisfied, not to the point at which you feel like your stomach is going to explode.

Q. There is a lot of protein on the 17 Day Diet? Why?

A: Protein is the major component of all of your body's cells, and it's important to make sure you're getting enough. Recent research indicates that we may need more than previously thought. According to the NHS, 15 per cent of your daily calories should come from protein. But you probably need more if you exercise, if you're dieting and as you age.

One dramatic study of 855 people found that those who ate just the RDA of protein had alarming bone losses compared to those who ate more than the RDA. Those who ate the least protein lost the most bone mass: 4 per cent in four years. People who ate the most protein (about 20 per cent of calories) had the smallest losses: less than 1.5 per cent in four years, reported the *Journal of Bone and Mineral Research* in 2000.

Although the study was done on older men and women, the results may be important for all adults. When you're young you need protein to build bone. After the age of 30, you need it to keep bone from being lost. Keeping bones strong is a life-long effort.

As for weight loss, take note: research keeps proving that a protein-dense diet is essential for weight loss. It helps maximise fat loss whilst minimising muscle loss. That's important because losing muscle slows your resting metabolic rate – the speed at which your body burns calories. That makes it harder to maintain a healthy weight and lose fat. By eating regularly from the foods on the 17 Day Diet lists, you'll get more than enough protein.

Q. I'm a vegetarian. Can I follow the 17 Day Diet?

A. Yes. If you're a 'lacto-ovo-vegetarian', you limit your protein to dairy products and eggs. That means you'll obtain your protein from probiotics such as yoghurt, eggs and beans and pulses (depending on which Cycle you're on). 'Semi-vegetarians', who avoid red meat but eat fish or chicken, can easily follow the diet. 'Vegans' avoid all animal proteins. If you're a vegan, you can still follow the diet. Simply use vegan meat substitutes at meals for protein and use a probiotic supplement in place of yoghurt. The 17 Day Diet adapts to virtually any nutritional lifestyle.

Q: I know that whole grains are really good for me, but I get bored with porridge and brown rice. What are some other ones I can try?

A. There are plenty of other choices. Look into some of the so-called ancient or alternative grains: amaranth (high in protein), kamut (a cousin of wheat), quinoa (a grain-like herb), spelt (a relative of wheat), triticale (a cross between rye and wheat, wholegrain risotto (a delicious type of rice), barley (super-high in fibre) and bulgar (a delicious form of wheat). To find some of these more uncommon grains, you may need to make a trip to a natural health shop or local ethnic food market. Many are unfamiliar to Westerners but have been eaten in other parts of the world for thousands of years.

Q. Sometimes I can't eat all the food allowed on the 17 Day Diet. Will this interfere with my results?

A. No, not at all. The 17 Day Diet is very filling. For many people it's a challenge to eat all those fruits and vegetables for the first time. If you can't eat all the food, don't worry about it. Just don't substitute those foods with foods not on the diet.

Q. I overindulged all weekend. What do you suggest?

A. If you gained 1.4 to 2.25 kg (3 to 5 lb) over the weekend, I advise that you go right back to Accelerate (Cycle 1) until you lose that weight. After that, continue on with the other Cycles to reach your goal weight.

Nutrition Questions

Q. Is it better to choose organic foods?

A. These days, we need to find out where everything comes from and how it's been grown or raised. Is it organic, cage-free, free-range or was it just grown in someone's back garden? We do need to reduce our exposure to toxins, or else they get stored in our body's fat cells. Scientists think this build-up of toxins may prevent weight loss. So buy organic whenever you can. Eating organic foods helps you naturally rid your body of toxins. Because some produce contains more pesticides than others, try to choose organic when shopping for these fruits and veggies: apples, nectarines, peaches, pears, strawberries, raspberries, cherries, grapes, peppers, celery, potatoes and spinach.

Q. What is your recommendation on taking a standard multivitamin?

A. I'm in favour of it. Taking vitamins and other supplements is important, but it can take quite a bit of time to pop everything you need. You may require a multiple vitamin and mineral, omega-3 fatty acids to reduce inflammation, calcium for bones and vitamin D.

Multivitamins can be especially helpful for anyone who doesn't eat a healthy diet or eat enough 'good' foods to obtain the vitamins we need for sustained good health. Plus as we age our bodies don't absorb certain vitamins such as vitamin B12 as well as they once did. We also need more vitamin D and calcium, but those can be consumed in separate supplements and not necessarily part of a multivitamin.

If you feel a multivitamin is important to your health, take a bottle of vitamins to your doctor to make sure the doses are safe (mega-doses of some vitamins can be dangerous), and make sure that there are no potential inter-actions between the vitamin supplements and any medicines you're taking.

Q. You recommend a natural low-calorie sweetener. What is it?

A. Shop about in health-food shops. One that is available in the US and expected to be available in the UK is Truvia. It is derived from stevia, a plant found in South America and Asia. This means that it is neither a sugar nor a purely artificial sweetener, but is instead a 'natural' zero-calorie sweetener. Truvia also contains erythritol, a kind of sugar alcohol found in fruits. As sugar substitutes go, Truvia is probably better than some lab-produced artificial sweeteners, which is why I recommend it. You can also cook and bake with Truvia. But like anything else, use it in moderation

Q. Can I use other sugar substitutes on the 17 Day Diet?

A. Artificial sweeteners are found in many foods these days, such as reduced-sugar yoghurt, which is one of the recommended probiotics on the 17 Day Diet. Clinically speaking, all sugar substitutes are testing safely; we just don't know much about their long-term health effects.

Six of the most common sugar substitutes currently available are aspartame (Equal), saccharine, acesulfame K, sucralose (Splenda), sugar alcohols and in the US stevia (Truvia and Sweet Leaf). Aspartame, saccharine, acesulfame K and sucralose are all chemical sugar substitutes that do provide some health benefits: they are lower in calories than regular sugar, and they do not raise blood sugar, particularly helpful for people with diabetes. Nor do these sweeteners promote tooth decay.

Sugar alcohols, such as mannitol and xylitol, are carbohydrates but not sugars, which make them sugar-free sweeteners. Unlike artificial sweeteners they can raise blood sugar, but because they are slowly absorbed from the intestinal tract, the rise in blood glucose and demand for insulin is minimal compared to eating pure sugar. They too are low calorie compared to natural sugar and do not promote tooth decay. Stevia (see above) is a newer artificial sweetener which is a natural extract from the stevia plant.

My advice is to go easy on sugar substitutes and learn to enjoy the natural sweetness of fresh fruits.

Q. I am trying to kick my sodium habit. Do you have any suggestions?

A. You might start by using a reduced-sodium salt alternative to wean yourself off sodium. Start cooking with herbs and spices too, especially garlic powder and onion powder to season meat or vegetables.

When buying ready-prepared foods, purchase reduced-sodium versions. Buy and use the sodium-free marinades for chicken, beef, pork and seafood.

When buying and using canned vegetables and beans, rinse them under running water at home. This will remove up to 40 per cent of the sodium. Or buy beans canned in water with no added salt.

The taste for salt is a learnt habit. Just as you acquired a taste for salty foods, you can also become accustomed to less salt.

Q: I've been hearing more and more about the health benefits of coffee and tea. But they both have caffeine, right? Which has more?

A: The fact that coffee and tea are good for you isn't new. The first written records of coffee from about 1000 years ago mention it as a medicine. Over the years herbalists have thought it could treat head and muscle aches, asthma and fatigue. Early references to tea in China involve boiling raw, wild tea leaves in water to soothe respiratory infections.

You already know that the caffeine in your morning cup of coffee keeps you alert and active. Now the Harvard Nurses' Health Study, a long-term examination of the habits of more than 100,000 nurses, has shown that there is a decreased risk of developing type 2 diabetes amongst participants who regularly drink coffee (caffeinated or decaf). Coffee is terrifically high in antioxidants, along with minerals such as potassium and magnesium and the B vitamins. All of these nutrients might be the reason coffee guards against type 2 diabetes.

The good coffee news just keeps on coming: research linked regular coffee consumption (three to four cups per day) to a decrease in the incidence of Parkinson's disease. Scientists have found that even an extra espresso may even help stave off mental decline as you age, according to a 2002 study published in the *American Journal of Epidemiology*.

So grab a cup of coffee, sink into an oversized chair and read the next question.

Q. If coffee and tea are so good for us, should I drink more?

A. Well, too much of any good thing becomes not such a good thing. How much you consume depends on your health and your caffeine tolerance. Most doctors say three to four 240 ml (8 fl oz) cups of caffeinated coffee or tea is the maximum that an individual should have daily.

Be aware that caffeine stimulates the central nervous and cardiovascular systems and is a diuretic. Too much coffee or tea can result in elevated blood pressure, insomnia, nervousness or rapid, uncomfortable breathing. Also, tannins found in coffee and tea may decrease your ability to absorb iron. Drink your tea or coffee at least one hour before meals so you can digest the tannins before iron is released in your system.

Q. I keep hearing people knock high-fructose corn syrup. What is it exactly? And is it really bad for you?

A: High-fructose corn syrup (HFCS) is the American term for glucose-fructose syrup, which can be found on the labels of many UK products such as fizzy drinks and squash, ice cream, flavoured yoghurts, cakes and pastries and even cough medicines. It is a potent sweetener made from corn starch. It's actually twice as sweet as sugar. Manufacturers began using it as a cheap sugar substitute in the 1970s when the price of sugar shot up. HFCS now accounts for 40 per cent of the caloric sweeteners added to foods and drinks.

Figures are not available in the UK, but Americans down about 132 calories' worth of HFCS a day, mainly in fizzy drinks and squash. That's a lot. By simply slashing 132 calories daily, you can lose about 6 kg (13 lb) a year without doing anything else. But calories aren't the real concern with HFCS. This is: it seems to make us eat more in two ways. First, when soda manufacturers switched from sugar to HFCS, they used the same quantity by volume, so sodas today are much sweeter than they were 30 years ago. Regular exposure to their intense sweetness can make you crave other sweet foods too.

Second, your body metabolises HFCS differently. Unlike other sweeteners, HFCS doesn't produce a normal rise in insulin after a meal, which in turn reduces the usual levels of a hormone called leptin. Leptin makes you feel full so you stop eating. Too little leptin, and you'll eat too much. From everything I've read, I don't like HFCS and recommend avoiding it.

Q. I've heard over and over again that trans fat is bad for us. What I'm not sure of is what it is. And why is it bad?

A. Trans fat is formed when unsaturated oils are put through a chemical process called hydrogenation. This process solidifies the oils at room temperature: think margarine or vegetable fat. Hard fat is needed to achieve specific characteristics in certain foods. For example, without a hard fat, biscuits would be soft, pie pastries would lose their flakiness and foods would go rancid more quickly.

Not all hard fats are trans fats though; some are saturated fats (the kind found in butter and cocoa butter, palm and coconut oils). But several years ago, the food industry moved away from using saturated fat because of its association with increased LDL ('lousy' cholesterol) levels. In making this switch the industry unknowingly created a fat that has turned out to be even worse for health: trans fat. In recent years, scientists have discovered that trans fatty acids not only raise LDL levels, they lower HDL ('good' cholesterol) – increasing your risk factors for heart disease. They also increase obesity.

Fortunately, fewer products are being manufactured with trans fats. If you're worried about whether a product contains trans fat, look on the ingredients label for the term 'partially hydrogenated'. Partially hydrogenated oil is trans fat.

Q. Are imitation seafood products good choices?

A. Imitation crab, prawns and other seafood (surimi) are usually made from Alaskan pollock, a white fish. The skinless, boneless fish is ground up, mixed with binders, salt and other flavours, cooked and then shaped. This imitation shellfish is an excellent source of low-fat protein and is lower in cholesterol than true shellfish.

A disadvantage is that it can contain nearly 700 milligrams of sodium in a modest 85 g (3 oz) portion. That's almost a third of the sodium limit recommended for a whole day and almost half of the limit recommended for people with sodium-sensitive high blood pressure.

Imitation seafood tastes pretty good. But if you don't like to eat anything 'fake', or with ingredients that sound unnatural, stick to the real deal.

Q. Every year I resolve to eat healthily, and I do – for two weeks or a month. How can I keep from falling back into my old diet patterns every year?

A. First of all keep making resolutions. The scientific literature shows that people who resolve to stop smoking, lose weight or start an exercise programme are much more likely to succeed than people who don't make resolutions.

Second, take action. Sitting around, thinking about change and talking about it doesn't make a difference. What produces change is action. Here are some action-oriented behaviours that are known to work for weight loss and prevent relapse:

- Eat breakfast every morning and regular, planned meals throughout the day.

- Exercise regularly. This concept is really simple – move it AND lose it.

- Guzzle more aqua. Water will really fill you up and assist in fat-burning.

- Start a love affair with veggies. Supplement your meals with healthy salads and veggies and make your mum proud.

* Eat before going to parties or other food-centred gatherings.

* Plan get-togethers with friends that don't revolve around food.

* Reward yourself for progress (but not with food), and ask friends and family members to do the same.

* In short set a goal – or resolution – plan concrete steps that will take you there, anticipate and avoid pitfalls, and reward yourself along the way.

Health Issues

Q. Just about everyone in my family is overweight. Is the deck stacked against me?

A. Yes, there is the genetic input to consider. People who research obesity discovered the 'blame-your-parents' factor. Their studies involved fat twins who were adopted by separate thin families. The twins remained heavy despite their slim surroundings. The study concluded that the ring around your middle, or at least some portion of it, comes from your parents, not just from what you eat when nobody is looking.

So yes, a family history of obesity may increase your odds of ending up overweight, but that just means you may have to work a little harder than those without such a history, to achieve and maintain a healthy weight. You're not doomed. In fact, researchers in the UK found that exercising can reduce the genetic tendency towards obesity by 40 per cent. Their findings were reported in *PLoS Medicine* in 2010. You can choose to adopt healthy habits. We inherit predispositions to certain problems, including obesity, but we also have the power to decide what to do about them.

Q. Does stress make people fat?

A. It appears there is some connection, and it's based on the theory of the 'caveman paunch'. It has to do with where fat settles in the body, and it goes something like this. Guys get beer bellies for the same reason women get thunder-thighs: it's a product of evolution. Cavewomen laid down stores of fat in their thighs and breasts to cope with the demands of pregnancy in the wild.

In cavemen flight-or-fight energy was stored as belly fat. When cavemen went beast-hunting and suddenly ended up being the hunted, their guts dispersed the fuel (fat) their muscles needed to run to safety. Since cavemen spent a lot of time fleeing, they never had much of a weight problem.

Nowadays, however, our predators are bosses, telephone sales people and issuers of credit cards. They are irritating, and it's hard to get away from them. A good idea is to lace up your trainers and go for a brisk walk. It's like hunting beasts but without any weapons. Regular exercise, seriously, really does prevent stress fat, plus a lot of other things.

Q. I'm a smoker. I know I should stop. But I'm afraid I'll gain weight. What do you think?

A. Let me ask you some questions: are you sacrificing what might help your health in the name of keeping off a few pounds? Where is your common sense? You might be surprised to learn that if you exercise whilst stopping smoking, you won't gain weight.

Exercising to get fit will also help you kick your cigarette habit. An Austrian study found that after three months, 80 per cent of smokers who did a cardio and strength-training workout three times a week whilst using a nicotine-replacement therapy of their choice (such as a patch, gum, an inhaler or a combination of them) had given up smoking; only 52 per cent of those who used nicotine replacement alone were successful. Plus, unlike such tools as prescription medications, exercise has no negative side effects. Take a cue from the research lab and walk, cycle and jog your way to a smoke-free and strong, fit body. Confer with your doctor about your exercise regime as you wean yourself off tobacco.

Q. I'm 56, and I've recently been diagnosed with pre-diabetes. What kind of screening tests should I have, and what should I do to help make sure it doesn't progress to diabetes?

A. Pre-diabetes is when a person's blood glucose levels are higher than normal, but not high enough for a diabetes diagnosis. If you are pre-diabetic, you have a substantially increased risk of heart attack, stroke, cancer, kidney disease, blindness, nerve damage and several other serious conditions.

Given your recent diagnosis of pre-diabetes, your doctor may recommend you follow certain lifestyle modifications such as diet, exercise and weight loss. There are several things you can do to help treat pre-diabetes and prevent the onset of type 2:

* **Eat a healthy diet and lose weight:** Losing only 5 to 7 per cent of your current body weight can usually bring the blood sugar down to normal ranges.

* **Exercise:** Get at least 30 minutes of activity a day, five days a week. Fat blunts insulin's ability to lower blood sugar. With less fat on board, your blood sugar can normalise.

* **Treat high blood pressure and cholesterol:** If you have been told that you have either of these conditions, speak to your doctor on the best course of treatment to get them in check.

* **Stop smoking:** Diabetes is not the only reason to stop, as smoking contributes to many other health problems.

* **Educate yourself:** Education is key for pre-diabetes and type 2 diabetes management. Diabetes is a complex condition and needs close monitoring to help you remain as active and healthy as possible. Doctors are very helpful in assisting any newly diagnosed patient with diabetes management. You can also contact Diabetes UK, a charity for people with diabetes.

Q. What are the best foods for my joints?

A. If your joints hurt, they might be inflamed. But taking painkillers isn't the only way to stop the pain. You can eat your way to more comfort with a fresh, unprocessed diet, as I suggest on the 17 Day Diet. Try eating fish such as sardines, wild salmon or white fish, such as cod or pollack, at least twice per week. Include daily servings of wholegrains and pulses, fruits (particularly berries) and vegetables – basically all the foods that are a part of the 17 Day Diet. These will give you the vitamins and minerals, omega-3 fatty acids and other nutrients you need to protect cells from inflammation.

Another common yet generally safe remedy is glucosamine, available as a supplement. Many people get relief from taking it. Consult your doctor about whether to take it, which kind to take and how much.

Q. My HDL cholesterol is low. What can I do to raise it?

A. Weight control and regular physical activity are the most important steps you can take to raise your 'good' HDL cholesterol. Higher HDL levels are linked with lower risk of heart disease, whilst low HDL is considered a major cardiovascular risk factor and is now being linked with greater risk of memory loss later in life. Low HDL levels are often associated with being overweight, especially if excess body fat is congregating at the waistline.

Studies suggest that overweight people who reach and maintain a healthier weight may raise low HDL levels anywhere from 5 to 20 per cent. Daily moderate aerobic physical activity such as walking or swimming is also very effective at raising low HDL. Although some people assume a low-fat diet is beneficial, completely cutting out heart-healthy fat (such as olive oil or omega-3 fats) can hurt rather than help your efforts. In addition, it's important to avoid smoking, which is linked with lower HDL, and to make sure that blood sugar is under control.

Genetics play a role in your HDL levels, and it's hard to change genetics. But with diet and exercise, you have two breakthrough tools to help you increase your HDL. Both are really the best medicine – and safe and cheap too!

Q. Are there foods I can eat for better skin?

A. Yes. Foods rich in 'beauty nutrients' can make your skin clearer, smoother and more radiant. Salmon is an excellent source of omega-3 fatty acids, which lubricate skin from within and prevent acne; kiwi fruits and blueberries provide vitamin C, which helps prevent wrinkles; oysters are rich in zinc, crucial for collagen production and sweet potatoes and tomatoes contain carotenoids, which may protect skin against damaging UV rays.

Q. Can people who are already overweight reduce their cancer risk if they lose weight?

A. The NHS states that amongst non-smokers, obesity is the most important preventable risk factor for cancer. In other words, if you don't smoke (which has the highest link to cancer), not being obese is the most important way to reduce your risk of cancer. Many adult cancers develop over a 10- to 20-year period or longer. Although researchers can't say for sure that losing weight will lower cancer risk, there is evidence that is looking promising. For example, two large studies of post-menopausal women found that those who lost weight after menopause reduced their risk of breast cancer substantially.

When overweight people lose weight, they may not be able to undo cancer-causing damage that's already done, but shedding excess fat can reduce elevated levels of insulin, insulin-related growth factors and certain hormones such as oestrogen. All these compounds are associated with the process of cancer development. Each loss or gain of excess body fat seems to change cancer risk.

Q. Is it true that sugar 'feeds' cancer?

A. While all cells in our body use sugar (glucose) for fuel, research does suggest that cancer cells take up blood sugar more rapidly than healthy cells. In addition, high blood sugar stimulates increased levels of insulin in our body, which may promote the growth of cancer cells.

Although this may sound frightening, the answer is not to avoid all sugar-containing foods. The sugar in our bloodstream comes from all carbohydrate foods, including vegetables, fruits, whole grains and low-fat dairy sources; some glucose is even produced within our bodies from protein.

For now our best answer is to keep blood sugar controlled with weight maintenance, regular exercise and a high-fibre diet. It's also important to avoid big loads of carbohydrate at once, particularly from refined grains such as white bread or foods with added sugars. Hopefully, further research will provide more answers.

Food Allergies

Q. An allergist told me recently I suffer from lactose intolerance. What can be done about this, as I find it hard to face a life without dairy products?

A. Lactose intolerance, is not an allergy but is caused by a lack of one or more enzymes that digest lactose, the carbohydrate in milk. Symptoms are bloating, diarrhoea, wind, nausea and abdominal cramps. Unfortunately, the recommended treatment is a lactose-free diet. If you avoid all dairy products you should also take calcium supplements. You can also buy lactase drops or tablets that can help you digest dairy products if taken before eating them. And lactose-free milk and cheese are available in supermarkets. If you're lactose intolerant, you'll likely find yoghurt much more digestible than milk. That's because those friendly bacteria digest some of the milk sugar in yoghurt, so there's less left to irritate you. You shouldn't have any trouble following the 17 Day Diet with this food sensitivity.

Q. I have to be on a gluten-free diet. Which foods are naturally gluten-free?

A. For background, about one out of 100 people in the UK has coeliac disease, an auto-immune intestinal disorder that causes severe allergies to proteins found in wheat and related grains. Even more people are gluten intolerant. For people with severe allergies to gluten, it's the difference between life and death, and a gluten-free diet is the only means of treatment. It prevents the complications of untreated coeliac disease, such as osteoporosis, anaemia, certain forms of cancer and even death. For people with intolerances to gluten, the benefits of a gluten-free diet are many: fewer sinus infections, more energy, less brain fog or less gastrointestinal upset. Some people lose weight on a gluten-free diet, but that may be because many high-calorie foods contain wheat, which is a carbohydrate:

Here is partial list of gluten-free foods:

* Milk (non-fat milk powder)
* 100 per cent vegetable juices
* Fresh fruits and vegetables that are not coated with a wax or resin that contains gluten
* A variety of single-ingredient foods: eggs, lentils, seeds such as flax, tree nuts such as almonds, no gluten-containing grains such as maize, meats, fresh fish and fresh shellfish
* Gluten-free foods such as bread, pastas and special cereals

Foods that are not gluten-free include:

* Barley, common wheat, rye, spelt, kamut, triticale
* Farina, vital gluten, semolina, malt vinegar

As for oats, no one agrees yet whether people with coeliac disease can eat them or not. Research data suggests that the majority of people with coeliac disease can tolerate a daily intake of a limited amount (e.g., 55 g/2 oz) of oats that are free of gluten from wheat, rye, barley or their crossbred hybrids.

By the way, if you're on a gluten-free diet, you can easily follow the 17 Day Diet by making food substitutions to include gluten-free products.

Keep those cards and letters coming... and visit me on the 17 Day website, www.the17daydiet.com, for more help and advice on how to live the diet and stay healthy and fit.

Resources

• • • • • • • • • • • •

Much of the material in this book comes from computer searches of medical databases of abstracts, medical news reports in both popular and specialised publications, as well as published scientific reports in peer-reviewed journals.

Chapter 1: Just Give Me 17 Days

Nackers, L.M., et al. 2010. The association between rate of initial weight loss and long-term success in obesity treatment: does slow and steady win the race? *International Journal of Behavioral Medicine* 17:161–167.

Laaksonen D., E., et. al. 2003. Relationships between changes in abdominal fat distribution and insulin sensitivity during a very low calorie diet in abdominally obese men and women. *Nutrition, Metabolism, and Cardiovascular Diseases* 13:349–356.

Leigh, Gibson E., and Green, M.W. 2002. Nutritional influences on cognitive function: mechanisms of susceptibility. *Nutrition Research Reviews* 15:169–206.

Bui, C., 2010. Acute effect of a single high-fat meal on forearm blood flow, blood pressure and heart rate in healthy male Asians and Caucasians: a pilot study. *The Southeast Asia Journal of Tropical Health and Public Health* 41:490–500.

Rudkowska, I., et. al. 2008. Cholesterol-lowering efficacy of plant sterols in low-fat yoghurt consumed as a snack or with a meal. *Journal of the American College of Nutrition* 27:588–595.

Johnston, C.S., 2002. Postprandial thermogenesis is increased 100% on a high-protein, low-fat diet versus a high-carbohydrate, low-fat diet in healthy, young women. *Journal of the American College of Nutrition* 21:55–61.

Hanninen, O., et. al. 1992. Effects of eating an uncooked vegetable diet for one week. Appetite 19:243–254.

Nowson, C.A., 2003. Dietary approaches to reduce blood pressure in a community setting: a randomised crossover study. *Asia Pacific Journal of Clinical Nutrition* 12 Suppl:S19.

Jenkins, D.J., et. al. 2009. The effect of a plant-based low-carbohydrate ('Eco-Atkins') diet on body weight and blood lipid concentrations in hyperlipidemic subjects. *Archives of Internal Medicine* 169:1046–1054.

Henkin, Y., and Shai, I. 2003. Dietary treatment of hypercholesterolemia: can we predict long-term success? *Journal of the American College of Nutrition* 22:555–561.

Kiortsis, D.N. et. al. 2001 Changes in lipoprotein(a) levels and hormonal correlations during a weight reduction programme. *Nutrition, Metabolism, and Cardiovascular Diseases* 11:153–157.

Claessens M., et. al. 2009. The effect of a low-fat, high-protein or high-carbohydrate ad libitum diet on weight loss maintenance and metabolic risk factors. *International Journal of Obesity* 33:296–304.

Janiszewski, P.M., and Ross, R. 2010. Effects of weight loss among metabolically healthy obese men and women. *Diabetes Care* 33:1957–1959.

Sheets, V., and Ajmere, K. 2005. Are romantic partners a source of college students' weight concern? *Eating Behaviors* 6:1–9.

Binks, M. 2005. Duke study reports sex, self-esteem diminish for morbidly obese. *CDS Review* 98(4):28–29.

Lapidus, L. 1984. Distribution of adipose tissue and risk of cardiovascular disease and death: a 12-year follow up of participants in the population study of women in Gothenburg, Sweden. *British Medical Journal* 289:1257.

Tran, T.T. 2008. Beneficial effects of subcutaneous fat transplantation on metabolism. *Cell Metabolism* 7:410–420.

Gunn, D.A. 2009. Why some women look young for their age. *PLoS One* 4:e8021.

Maconochie, N. 2007. Risk factors for first trimester miscarriage – results from a UK-population-based case-control study. *BJOG* 114:170–186.

Chapter 2: Burn, Baby, Burn

McCrory M.,A., et. al. 1999. Dietary variety within food groups: association with energy intake and body fatness in men and women. *American Journal of Clinical Nutrition* 69:440–447.

Pataky, Z. 2009 Gut microbiota, responsible for our body weight? *Revue Medicale Suisse* 5:662–664, 666.

Scarpellini, E. 2010. Gut microbiota and obesity. *Internal and Emergency Medicine* 5 Suppl 1:S53–56.

Diamant, M., 2010. Do nutrient-gut-microbiota interactions play a role in human obesity, insulin resistance and type 2 diabetes? *Obesity Review*, August 13.

Kim, D.H., et al. 2010. Peptide designed to elicit apoptosis in adipose tissue endothelium reduces food intake and body weight. *Diabetes* 59:907–915.

Yang, C.S., and Wang, X. 2010. Green tea and cancer prevention. *Nutrition and Cancer* 62(7):931–937.

Chapter 3: Cycle 1: Accelerate

Tremblay, A., et al. 2004. Thermogenesis and weight loss in obese individuals: a primary association with organochlorine pollution. *International Journal of Obesity and Related Metabolic Disorders* 28(7):936–939.

Chapter 4: Cycle 2: Activate

Varady, K.A. 2007. Alternate-day fasting and chronic disease prevention: a review of human and animal trials. *American Journal of Clinical Nutrition* 86:7–13.

Jakulj, F. 2007. A high-fat meal increases cardiovascular reactivity to psychological stress in healthy young adults. *Journal of Nutrition* 137:935–939.

Westerterp-Planteng, M.S., et. al. 2005. Sensory and gastrointestinal satiety effects of capsaicin on food intake. *International Journal of Obesity* 29:682–688.

Liu, H. 2010. Fructose induces transketolase flux to promote pancreatic cancer growth. *Cancer Research* 70:6368–6376.

Chapter 5: Cycle 3: Achieve

Di Blasio, A. 2010. Effects of the time of day of walking on dietary behaviour, body composition and aerobic fitness in post-menopausal women. *The Journal of Sports Medicine and Physical Fitness* 50:196–201.

Fischer-Posovszky, P. 2010. Resveratrol regulates human adipocyte number and function in a Sirt1-dependent manner. *American Journal of Clinical Nutrition* 92:5–15.

Fuchs, N. K. 2002. Liposuction lowers cholesterol. *Women's Health Letter*. Soundview Publications.

Vgontzas, A.N. 2007. Daytime napping after a night of sleep loss decreases sleepiness, improves performance and causes beneficial changes in cortisol and interleukin-6 secretion *American Journal of Physiology, Endocrinology, and Metabolism* 292: E253–E261.

National Weight Control Registry. www.nwcr.ws/Research/default.htm.

Rolls, B.J., et. al. 2004. Salad and satiety: energy density and portion size of a first-course salad affect energy intake at lunch. *Journal of the American Dietetic Association* 104:1570–1576.

Kristal, A.R. 2005. Yoga practice is associated with attenuated weight gain in healthy, middle-aged men and women. *Alternative Therapies in Health and Medicine* 11:28–33.

Chapter 8: The PMS Exception Diet

Hibbeln, J.R. 1998, Fish consumption and major depression. *The Lancet* 351:1213.

Hibbeln, J.R., and Salem, N. 1995. Dietary polyunsaturated fatty acids and depression: when cholesterol does not satisfy. *American Journal of Clinical Nutrition* 62: 1–9.

Benton, D., Cook, R. 1991. The impact of selenium supplementation on mood. *Biological Psychiatry* 29:1092–1098.

Hawkes, W.C., and Hornbostel, L. 1996. Effects of dietary selenium on mood in healthy men living in a metabolic research unit. *Biological Psychiatry* 39:121–128.

Kalman, D., et al. 2009. A prospective, randomised, double-blind, placebo-controlled parallel-group dual site trial to evaluate the effects of a Bacillus coagulans-based product on functional intestinal gas symptoms. *BMC Gastroenterology* 18:85.

Ghanbari Z., et. al. 2009 Effects of calcium supplement therapy in women with premenstrual syndrome. *Taiwan Journal Obstetrics and Gynecology* 48:124–129.

Chapter 10: Family Challenges

Paisley J, et. al. 2008. Dietary change: what are the responses and roles of significant others? *Journal of Nutrition Education and Behavior* 40:80–88.

Wallace, J.P. 1995. Twelve month adherence of adults who joined a fitness programme with a spouse versus without a spouse. *Journal of Sports Medicine and Physical Fitness* 35:206–213.

Morgan, D.V., et al. 1988. Mutual motivation. *Health*, August, 32–36.

Chapter 11: Surviving Holidays

Andersson, I., et. al. 1992. The Christmas factor in obesity therapy. *International Journal of Obesity and Related Metabolic Disorders* 16:013–1015.

Baker, R.C. et. al. Weight control during the holidays: Highly consistence self-monitoring as a potentially useful coping mechanism. *Health Psychology* 17:367–370.

Chapter 13: Shift Work on the 17 Day Diet

Geliebter, A. 2000. Work-shift period and weight change. *Nutrition* 16:27–29.

Henderson, N.J., and Christopher D.B.B. 1998. An evaluation of the effectiveness of shift work preparation strategies. *New Zealand Journal of Psychology*. New Zealand Psychological Society.

Thorpy, M.J. 2010. Managing the patient with shift-work disorder. *The Journal of Family Practice* 59(1 Suppl):S24–31.

Chapter 15: Doctor, Can You Please Tell Me More?

Marian, T. et al. 2000. Effect of dietary protein on bone loss in elderly men and women: The Framingham Osteoporosis Study. *Journal of Bone and Mineral Research* 15:2504–2512.

van Dam, R.M., et al. 2006. Coffee, caffeine and risk of type 2 diabetes: a prospective cohort study in younger and middle-aged U.S. women. *Diabetes Care* 29:398–403.

Checkoway H., et. al. 2002. Parkinson's disease risks associated with cigarette smoking, alcohol consumption and caffeine intake. *American Journal of Epidemiology*. 155:732–738.

Shengxu L., et al. 2010. Physical activity attenuates the genetic predisposition to obesity in 20,000 men and women from EPIC-Norfolk prospective population study. *PloS Medicine* e1000332. doi:10.1371/journal.pmed.1000332.

Shape Magazine. 2007. Trying to quit smoking? Get moving. Author.